Summer Incidents and Accidents

Editor

STEPHEN D. KRAU

CRITICAL CARE NURSING CLINICS OF NORTH AMERICA

www.ccnursing.theclinics.com

Consulting Editor
JAN FOSTER

June 2013 • Volume 25 • Number 2

ELSEVIER

1600 John F. Kennedy Boulevard • Suite 1800 • Philadelphia, Pennsylvania, 19103-2899

http://www.theclinics.com

CRITICAL CARE NURSING CLINICS OF NORTH AMERICA Volume 25, Number 2
June 2013 ISSN 0899-5885, ISBN-13: 978-1-4557-7078-6

Editor: Katie Saunders
Developmental Editor: Donald Mumford

Critical Care Nursing Clinics of North America (ISSN 0899-5885) is published quarterly by Elsevier Inc., 360 Park Avenue South, New York, NY 10010-1710. Months of issue are March, June, September, and December. Business and Editorial Offices: 1600 John F. Kennedy Blvd., Suite 1800, Philadelphia, PA 19103-2899. Periodicals postage paid at New York, NY and additional mailing offices. Subscription prices are $144.00 per year for US individuals, $308.00 per year for US institutions, $76.00 per year for US students and residents, $192.00 per year for Canadian individuals, $385.00 per year for Canadian institutions, $219.00 per year for international individuals, $385.00 per year for international institutions and $111.00 per year for Canadian and foreign students/residents. To receive student/resident rate, orders must be accompanied by name of affiliated institution, data of term, and the *signature* of program/residency coordinator on institution letterhead. Orders will be billed at individual rate until proof of status is received. Foreign air speed delivery is included in all *Clinics* subscription prices. All prices are subject to change without notice. **POSTMASTER:** Send address changes to *Critical Care Nursing Clinics of North America*, Elsevier Health Sciences Division, Subscription Customer Service, 3251 Riverport Lane, Maryland Heights, MO 63043. **Customer Service: 1-800-654-2452 (US and Canada); 314-447-8871 (outside US and Canada). Fax: 314-447-8029. E-mail: JournalsCustomerService-usa@elsevier.com (for print support) and JournalsOnlineSupport-usa@elsevier.com (for online support).**

Reprints. For copies of 100 or more of articles in this publication, please contact the Commercial Reprints Department, Elsevier Inc., 360 Park Avenue South, New York, New York, 10010-1710; Tel.: (212) 633-3813, Fax: (212) 462-1935, and E-mail: reprints@elsevier.com.

Critical Care Nursing Clinics of North America is covered in *MEDLINE/PubMed (Index Medicus), International Nursing Index, Nursing Citation Index, Cumulative Index to Nursing and Allied Health Literature,* and *RNdex Top 100.*

Printed and bound by CPI Group (UK) Ltd, Croydon, CR0 4YY

Transferred to digital print 2012

Contributors

CONSULTING EDITOR

JAN FOSTER, PhD, RN, CNS
College of Nursing, Texas Woman's University, Houston, Texas

EDITOR

STEPHEN D. KRAU, PhD, RN, CNE
Associate Professor, School of Nursing, Vanderbilt University Medical Center, Nashville, Tennessee

AUTHORS

RICHARD B. ARBOUR, MSN, RN, CCRN, CNRN, CCNS, FAAN
Critical Care Clinical Nurse Specialist, Philadelphia, Pennsylvania; Clinical Faculty, LaSalle University and Holy Family University, Philadelphia, Pennsylvania

STEPHANIE N. BAKER, PharmD, BCPS
Department of Pharmacy Services, UK Health Care; Department of Pharmacy Practice and Science, University of Kentucky College of Pharmacy, Lexington, Kentucky

DEBORAH L. ELLISON, PhD(c), MSN, RN
Associate Professor, Austin Peay State University, Clarksville, Tennessee

FRANCISCA FARRAR, EdD, MSN, RN
Professor of Nursing, School of Nursing, Austin Peay State University, McCord, Clarksville, Tennessee

CHIP GRESHAM, MD, FACEM
Emergency Medicine Physician, Medical Toxicologist and Co-Director of Emergency Medicine Education, Middlemore Hospital, Auckland, New Zealand

KRISTEN HERSHEY, MSN, RN
Assistant Professor, Austin Peay State University, School of Nursing, Clarksville, Tennessee

STEPHEN D. KRAU, PhD, RN, CNE
Associate Professor, School of Nursing, Vanderbilt University Medical Center, Nashville, Tennessee

MARIA L. OVERSTREET, PhD, RN
Assistant Professor, Vanderbilt University School of Nursing, Nashville, Tennessee

BENJAMIN A. SMALLHEER, PhD, RN, ACNP-BC, CCRN
Assistant Professor of Nursing, Vanderbilt University School of Nursing; Acute Care Nurse Practitioner, Special Care/Rapid Response Team, St. Thomas Hospital, Nashville, Tennessee

K. MELISSA SMITH, DNP, MSN, ANP-BC
Instructor of Nursing, Vanderbilt University School of Nursing, Nashville, Tennessee

JOSHUA SQUIERS, PhD, MSN, ANP-BC AGACNP-BC
Instructor of Nursing and Anesthesiology, Coordinator: ACNP Intensivist Sub-specialty, Vanderbilt University School of Nursing, Nashville, Tennessee

RICHARD S. VETTER, MS
Research Associate, Department of Entomology, University of California, Riverside, Riverside, California; Division of Biological Sciences, San Bernardino County Museum, Redlands, California

KYLE A. WEANT, PharmD, BCPS
North Carolina Public Health Preparedness and Response, North Carolina Department of Health and Human Services, Raleigh, North Carolina

JENNIFER WILBECK, DNP, APRN, CEN
Associate Professor and FNP/ACNP-ED Program Coordinator, Vanderbilt University School of Nursing, Nashville, Tennessee

CAROL C. ZIEGLER, DNP, FNP, RN
Assistant Professor, Vanderbilt University School of Nursing, Nashville, Tennessee

Contents

Combined, snake and scorpion encounters result in more than 25,000 calls a year to poison centers. Although some similarities exist with respect to general signs of envenomation and treatment, specific nuances distinguish the medical care to be anticipated and therapies available. Regardless of geographic practice area, exposures will occur that may result in a significant envenomation. This article provides critical care nurses with fundamental knowledge of varied snake and scorpion envenomation presentations and treatments to assist in optimizing patient outcomes.

This article reviews the growing epidemic of West Nile virus (WNV), clinical manifestations of the 2 primary groups of WNV, diagnostic tests, critical nursing management, risk factors, and prevention of WNV. Critical care nursing management is based on symptom management and supportive therapy for neuroinvasive disease complications. Nursing management for complications such as altered level of consciousness, mechanical ventilator respiratory support, high fever, cerebral edema, increased intracranial pressure, seizures, and neuropsychiatric issues is outlined. Preventive measures for WNV, such as surveillance programs, personal protective measures, source reduction, mosquito programs, and vaccine development, are discussed.

In North America, spider envenomation is perceived to be a greater threat than in actuality; however, it still is a valid source of morbidity and, very rarely, mortality. Only 2 groups (widows, recluses) are medically important on this continent. Widow bites affect the neuromuscular junction, have minor dermatologic expression, and are treated with analgesics and antivenom. Recluse bites vary from mild, self-limiting rashes to extensive dermonecrosis. Recent awareness of methicillin-resistant *Staphylococcus aureus* as a ubiquitous cause of skin injury that is often mistaken as attributable to recluse bites has questioned the credence of spiders being the cause of idiopathic wounds.

Rabies is a devastating encephalitis caused by RNA viruses that use mammals as reservoirs. In the United States, most naturally acquired human cases have come from bats. The use of appropriate preexposure and postexposure prophylaxis can be nearly 100% effective. If prophylaxis is not used, or is implemented incorrectly, the patient may develop clinical rabies, which is almost universally fatal. All health care practitioners should be familiar with the appropriate evaluation of patients presenting with a possible rabies exposure and ensure that expeditious and appropriate prophylaxis is provided to help prevent the development of this lethal disease.

> With forecast trends predicting climate changes that will result in warmer weather globally, the potential for heat-related morbidities and mortality increases. Critical care nurses are uniquely poised to have an impact on the health care consequences of persons exposed to excessive ambient heat. The first step is a clearer understanding of ambient heat, heat conditions, and heat factors. This understanding combined with knowledge of persons at highest risk for heat-related mortality and morbidity can lead to interventions to ameliorate the prevalence and incidence of these incidents.

> With current predictions of climate change, the incidence of heat-related illnesses is projected to increase. Heat-related illnesses occur on a continuum from mild symptoms to fatalities. To prevent heat-related illnesses, nurses should have comprehension of persons at risk. Primary treatment of heat-related illness centers on cooling, but not overcooling, the patient. Heatstroke involves coagulopathies and cytokines, and can result in systemic inflammatory response syndrome and multiple organ dysfunction. Critical care nursing intervention requires more than effective cooling to support bodily processes that have been damaged or destroyed by the pathophysiology of heatstroke.

> Hypertrophic cardiomyopathy is a complex cardiovascular disorder particularly sensitive to environmental changes and physiologic stress. Warm weather and strenuous activity can be a dangerous combination for people that have hypertrophic cardiomyopathy. Often sudden cardiac death is the first symptom of the disorder. Thorough sports histories and physicals are important preventive measures and referrals to cardiovascular specialists should occur for any suspicion of cardiac abnormalities. Treatment of hypertrophic cardiomyopathy is focused on abating the natural clinical progression that includes sudden cardiac death, severe heart failure symptoms, and arrhythmias. Safe, effective delivery of care to the patient with hypertrophic cardiomyopathy requires a deep understanding of the complexities surrounding this precarious cardiac condition.

> Burns are a leading cause of accidental injury and death. The American Burn Association statistics from 2001 to 2010 show that 68% of burns happen at home, 44% are from fires/flames, and 60% to 70% happen to white men. Smoke inhalation is the leading cause of adult death caused by fires. A patient with a 78% total body surface area burn has a 50% chance of

survival. Burn injuries are described in terms of causative agents, depth, and severity. Crucial treatments for people with burns include assessment, stabilization, transfer to a burn unit, and fluid resuscitation.

Summer invites activities and sports that are unique to this time of year. Although safety is a priority, there are commonly accidents and incidents that occur while individuals are participating in these activities. The prevalence and incidence of several types of injuries and trauma related to water activities, camping, caving, backpacking, and hiking are discussed. Treatment of nonfatal drowning is discussed, along with the pathophysiologic process that must be corrected for optimal outcomes. Summer is a time for outdoor cooking, campfires, and the traditional Fourth of July firework pastimes, which can result in admissions to critical care areas.

Traumatic brain injury, which may be blunt or penetrating, begins altering intracranial physiology at the moment of impact as primary brain trauma. This article differentiates blunt versus penetrating brain trauma, primary versus secondary brain injury, and subsequent intracranial pathophysiology. Discussion and case study correlate intracranial pathophysiology and multisystem influences on evolving brain injury with mechanism-based interventions to modulate brain components (brain, blood, and cerebrospinal fluid volumes). The discussion also explores the effects of controlled ventilation, cardiopulmonary physiology, and global physiologic state on secondary injury, control of intracranial pressure, and recovery.

This article highlights 2 important complications of fracture: acute compartment syndrome and fat embolism syndrome (FES). FES is most commonly associated with long-bone and pelvic fracture, whereas acute compartment syndrome is often associated with tibia or forearm fracture. The onset of both of these complications may be difficult to assess in the nonverbal patient or in the patient with multiple trauma. Careful, serial assessment of the patient with fracture is necessary to recognize and treat these complications promptly. Early treatment and supportive care are crucial to positive outcomes for patients with complications of fracture.

Travel abroad for business and pleasure should be safe and meaningful for the traveler. To assure that safe experience, certain processes should be considered before travel. A thorough pretravel health assessment will offer patients and health care providers valuable information for anticipatory guidance before travel. The destination-based risk assessment will help determine the risks involved in travel to specific locations and guide in the development of contingency plans for all travelers, especially those with chronic conditions. Diseases are more prevalent overseas, and immunizations and vaccinations are all important considerations for persons traveling abroad.

CRITICAL CARE NURSING CLINICS OF NORTH AMERICA

Preface

Summer Incidents and Accidents

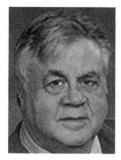

Stephen D. Krau, PhD, RN, CNE
Editor

The types of patients that we see in critical care are often a reflection of happenings that are occurring outside of the hospital walls. During natural disasters, such as hurricanes, tornadoes, and floods, it is not unusual to see patients who had succumbed or been injured during these disasters. Nonnatural disasters, such as multimotor vehicle accidents, disease outbreaks, and mass casualties of any sort, are also events that occur outside the hospital and impact the staff and resources of critical care units. Natural phenomena also impact the critical care unit census, and this would include seasonal changes.

The inspiration for this issue came from real clinical experiences that occurred one night in July a few years ago. Along with patients experiencing diabetic ketoacidosis, acute respiratory distress, and sepsis, there were several patients admitted with diagnoses that would most likely not be seen during this season. There were 2 snake bite patients, 1 spider bite patient, and a patient who had been transferred to our facility with Rocky Mountain spotted fever and heat stroke. While going to other critical care units that same week, I discovered that there were an abundance of patients with burns related to outdoor cooking and fireworks, and patients who endured accidents that interrupted their summer activities of pleasure.

This issue of *Critical Care Nursing Clinics of North America* is divided into 3 main sections. The first section centers on bites and stings; the second section is concentrated on heat and thermal injuries, and the third section focuses on traumatic events that commonly occur during summer months. The issue ends with an overview of recommendations for the critical care nurse as he or she considers his or her own summer travel, or cares for a patient who has just been abroad.

The issue starts with an overview of bites and stings. Although not all bites or stings are related to summer months, there are reproductive cycles and gathering cycles that

http://dx.doi.org/10.1016/j.ccell.2013.02.016
0899-5885/13/$ – see front matter © 2013 Published by Elsevier Inc.
ccnursing.theclinics.com

occur with many animals and insects that impact their aggressiveness and their visibility. It is important for the critical care nurse to review issues related to these bites, because they occur most frequently during the summer season. Articles on beestings, snake and spider bites, and tick-borne illnesses provide the reader with an overview and the latest information about diagnostics and treatment of the patient.

It is predicted that due to global climate change, the world will experience a higher number of heat waves with longer duration and more intensity than what we have experienced before.[1] This, along with a growing population, people with chronic medical conditions living longer, and our zeal for athletic pasttimes during summer months, contributes to the possibility of more heat-related illnesses being seen in our emergency departments and intensive care areas. This section discusses the heat-related illness continuum, thermal burns, and the phenomenon of hypertrophic cardiomyopathy, which has the potential to be more problematic in the presence of severe heat or dehydration.

The final section is devoted to accidents and trauma that may occur during any season, but are associated with many summer activities. Traumatic brain injuries as the result of many summer activities, along with fractures for the summer athlete and information, about global travel, are presented in the last section.

The articles chosen for this issue focus on events that are not limited to summer months but often occur during the summer. As seasonal changes occur, it may be months before seeing patients with these issues. Information about these phenomena and care for these patients may slip from the forefront of the nurse's mind. It is hoped that this issue of *Critical Care Nursing Clinics of North America* will serve as a "handbook" so to speak, with information to help the critical care nurse envision a broader perspective of the patient situation and to assist in the planning of optimal care.

Stephen D. Krau, PhD, RN, CNE
School of Nursing
Vanderbilt University Medical Center
461 21st Avenue South
309 Godchaux Hall
Nashville, TN 37240, USA

E-mail address:
steve.krau@vanerbilt.edu

REFERENCE

1. O'Neill MS, Carter R, Kish JK, et al. Preventing heat-related morbidity and mortality: new approaches to a changing climate. Maturitas 2009;64:98–103.

Bites and Stings
Epidemiology and Treatment

Stephen D. Krau, PhD, RN, CNE

KEYWORDS

- Bites • Stings • Dog bites • Cat bites • Summer bites • Bee stings

KEY POINTS

- Most bites and stings that are seen in hospital settings occur during the summer months.
- Although benign, many bites and stings can cause severe systemic conditions including fatalities if untreated.
- The time lapse between the actual bite and treatment is one of the stongest determinants of patient outcomes.
- Dog bites, bee stings, and cat bites are among the most prevalent bites that occur in the United States.
- Although rare, aquatic animal bites, spider bites, and scorpion bites can lead to fatalities through very different physiologic mechanisms.

BITES AND STINGS: EPIDEMIOLOGY AND TREATMENT: AN OVERVIEW

The adverse effects of stings and bites can range from minor skin irritation to lethal anaphylaxis, paralysis, and death. During the summer months, dogs, cats, insects, snakes, and spiders abound. Additionally, warmer weather induces hikers, swimmers, canoers, kayakers, and bikers to engage in summer time activities where animals habitate in the wild. Outdoor activities remove the home barrier of protection and expose people to elements, and all of the creatures that live in those elements. The realm of animal bites is quite extensive and complex and to suggest that all aspects can be considered in 1 manuscript is unreasonable. Herein is an overview of salient aspects of bites and stings.

CANINE BITES

Dog bites are the most common animal bite injuries in the United States, with an estimated infection rate between 15% and 20%.[1] Each year 800,000 Americans seek medical assistance for dog bites. The average mortality of dog bites is about 18 deaths per year.[2–4] Although German Shepherds account for 50% of the reported canine bites,

School of Nursing, Vanderbilt University Medical Center, 461 21st Avenue South, Nashville, TN 37240, USA
E-mail address: steve.krau@vanderbilt.edu

Crit Care Nurs Clin N Am 25 (2013) 143–150
http://dx.doi.org/10.1016/j.ccell.2013.02.008
0899-5885/13/$ – see front matter © 2013 Elsevier Inc. All rights reserved.

they rank third, and follow Pit Bulls and Rottweilers for dog bite-related fatalities.[5,6] Dog bite victims are most likely to be boys, with a peak incidence between 5 and 9 years of age.[7] Because of their small size, dog bites most commonly affect the face and neck of children. In adults, the bites are more likely to be on the extremities.

Injuries related to dog bites include the crushing tissue damage, deep puncture wounds, and exposure to underlying cartilage that occurs with the bite and the pulling of the victim by the dog when the bite occurs. These factors, along with a delay in seeking treatment beyond 6 to 12 hours can contribute to higher rates of wound infection.[7,8] There are a variety of bacterial pathogens associated with dog bites, with the most common aerobic isolates being *Staphylococcus* species, *Streptococcus* species, *Corynebacterium* species, *Moraxella* species, and *Neisseria* species.[5] Common anaerobes include *Bacteroides fragilis*, *Prevotella*, *Prophyromonas*, *Peptostreptococcus, and Fusobacterium*.[5,7] Recent consideration has been given to *Capnocytophagia canimorsus*, which is a gram-negative rod strongly associated with dog bites and known to cause life-threatening infections in people.[1] The appropriate use and selection of antibiotics should be based on the understanding that wound infections tend to be polymicrobial in nature.

In addition to bacterial wound infections, the critical care nurse must also consider the possibility of viral infections that have been transmitted from a dog bite. One of the more salient viruses transmitted by dogs is the rabies virus, in which dog bites worldwide account for 97% of human rabies cases.[9] In the United States due to animal control and vaccination programs, rabies is more likely to be transmitted from skunks, raccoons, bats, and foxes than they are from domestic dogs.[1] **Table 1** presents an overview of the assessment considerations and treatment standards involved in caring for a patient who has been the victim of a dog or cat bite.

CAT BITES

The frequency of dog bites as a mammalian source of bites is followed by cat bites. Studies have demonstrated that among mammalian bites, cat bites constitute about 12% to 25% of those bites, followed by bites from rodents and wild animals, which account for 4% of mammalian bites.[2,5,10–12] Cat bites victims are more commonly women, and of older age groups.[7] Additionally, cat bites are 2 times more likely to occur in the home environment as compared to dog bites.[2]

Compared with dog bites, cat bites present with higher rates of infection. Although data are somewhat limited, it is estimated that cat bite injuries manifest with infections in 30% to 50% of cases.[2,7] Additionally, signs of infection present much more rapidly (typically within 12 hours) when compared with dog bites.[5,7] Cats have long slender teeth that inoculate bacteria into deep tissues, and they also have unique feline flora in their mouths.[5,7,13]

The bacteria associated with cat bite wounds are similar to the bacteria discussed with dog bite wounds. One of the exceptions to this is the pathogen *Pasteurella multocida*. This pathogen is a major concern with cat bites and has been estimated to occur in 50% to 75% of cat bite infections.[5,7] Infections caused by *Pasteurella* demonstrate a rapid progression, and this agent has been identified as a causative agent in sepsis related to bite wounds.[14] **Table 1** describes the assessment and treatment of the bite victim, including the cat bite patient.

NON-CANINE BITES AND STINGS

There is support that the risk of being bitten by noncanine species is during greatest during summer months.[11,15] When considering bites and stings from all noncanine

Table 1
Clinical evaluation and treatment of animal bites

History	Information regarding the events of the bite should be ascertained:
	The type of animal, its behavior, ownership, and current immunization status
	The time of the injury and the time elapsed since the bite should be considered, as longer duration between the bite and seeking medical treatment increases the chance of infection
	Any relevant history related to wound healing should be obtained, including
	Any disease processes such as diabetes or human immunodeficiency virus that might inhibit wound healing
	Any conditions requiring long-term corticosteroid therapy or immunosuppression[5]
	Medication history and allergies should be documented
	The immunization status of the victim warrants attention.
Physical Examination	The location and extent of the bite injury should be considered along with any symptoms the patient reports
	Determine the type of wound as a puncture, laceration, avulsion, or crush injury, or any combination of these 4 main types
	The amount of the tissue affected and its location
	If fractures are suspected, radiographic studies should be included
	The wound should be examined for signs of infection and cultured if suspected
	Fresher wounds are not as likely to demonstrate signs of infection to the same extent those that have had a delay in treatment
	Other symptoms such as nausea, vomiting, and changes in mentation or visual acuity should be determined
	Blood cultures should be obtained if there is evidence of systemic toxicity or immunosuppression
Initial Wound Care	The goal is to achieve rapid healing, while minimizing infection risk and preserving optimal function and aesthetic quality
	Removal of any foreign bodies such as teeth or debris should be followed by proper cleansing.
	All wounds should be irrigated with at least 500 mL, normal saline at a pressure greater than 7 psi (18 gauge catheter on a 60 mL syringe).[5]
	Puncture wounds with inherent lack of drainage should be irrigated to allow the escape of fluid avoiding surrounding tissue hyrdrodissection and edema
	If a wound is markedly contaminated or infected, the use of an antiseptic irrigant is indicated
	Prior to closure of the wound, judicious debridement of devitalized or necrotic tissue should be completed along with maintaining clean wound edges to promote healing
Wound Exploration and Closure	The major risk of early closure of the wound is the possibility of infection
	Wound closure will be done based on the location of the wound and type of wound

(continued on next page)

Table 1 *(continued)*	
Antibiotics	The initiation of antibiotic therapy in the presence of obvious infection is a standard of care
	The choice of antibiotic is contingent upon the isolates found in the wound Antibiotic choice may change as culture results are determined
	The most effective single agent to cover pathogens associated with dog, cat, and human bites is oral amoxicillin and clavulanate
	If intravenous antibiotics are to be used, the most appropriate choices are ampicillin and sulbactam[5]
	The decision to initiate prophylactic antibiotics in uninfected dog bite wounds is controversial[5]
	There are not sufficient data to support evidence-based guidelines for prophylactic antibiotic therapy in uninfected wounds
	In cases of isolates of *C canimorsus*, due to its tendency to cause septic shock, there are strong recommendations to consider treating the patient with prophylactic antibiotics, especially is the patient is asplenic or uses alcohol
	Due to higher rates of infection in cat bites than in dog bite episodes, prophylactic antibiotics are commonly recommended for cat bites[5]
Postexposure Prophylaxis	Rabies: depends on biting species, local prevalence of the disease, availability of the animal for testing, and to what extent the bite was provoked—current guidelines available from the Centers for Disease Control and Prevention
	Tetanus: prophylaxis recommended if the patient has had fewer than 3 tetanus toxoid doses or more than 5 years have elapsed since the last immunization

sources, the crude rate of bite or sting injuries is about 316.6 bites/stings per 100.000 population per year.[15] An extensive national study reported that the most frequent bite or sting was an unspecified insect (39.2%), followed by bees (17.7%), then spiders (12.8%) and cats (7.3%). The study indicated that less than 1% of bee sting, 2.5% of spider bite, and 3.7% of cat bite victims were hospitalized.[15] Conversely, although rare, more than half of the victims of a venomous snake bite (58.4%) were hospitalized.[15]

Insects

Bees, wasps, and hornets are found throughout the United States and are most abundant in summer months.[16] Thousands of people are stung or bitten by insects each year, and in the United States as many as 90 to 100 people die as a result of allergic reactions.[16] Insects belonging to the order *Hymenoptera* constitute the majority of insects whose stings and bites cause most insect hypersensitivity reactions. These insects fall into 3 categories, which include *Formicidae* (fire ants), *Apidae* (honeybee and bumblebees), and *Vespidade* (hornets, yellow jackets, and wasps).[17]

In recent years, bumblebees have become an important etiology of sting reactions in many settings, including occupational settings. The venom of the bumblebee is different from the venom of honeybees. This requires different allergy testing. To date, there is no approved diagnostic testing or treatment of bumblebee allergy in the United States.[17]

Acute treatment

Recent guidelines emphasize the role of early recognition and prevention of insect sting-induced anaphylaxis and the early administration of epinephrine.[17] The use of epinephrine has been the source of some controversy, as there are indications that epinephrine is underutilized in emergency settings.[18–20] Even in situations where the patient has comorbidities such as hypertension, cardiac arrhythmias, or the use of concomitant medications, epinephrine should be used. As anaphylaxis can be fatal, delays in administration can result in patient mortality, and there are no contraindications for its use in life-threatening situations.[17,20] It is still the preferred practice that patients who have experience a systemic reaction to a sting carry an injectable device to use in the event of a subsequent bite. It is also recommended that patients might require more than 1 injection of epinephrine to prevent anaphylaxis and that more than 1 device be prescribed.[21] Although epinephrine injection devices are not typically required for persons at low risk for anaphylaxis, the decision whether to carry an injectable epinephrine should be made following discussions with the patient and primary care provider.

SNAKES

The actual incidence of snake bites worldwide is thought to be underestimated, because in many parts of the world, bite victims are treated by traditional healers and go unreported. Epidemiologic studies in Asia and Africa have demonstrated that there are 4 to 162 snake bite deaths annually per 100,000 people.[22] Bites from snakes in the United States have seasonal variations, with summer being a peak due to outdoor activities as well as occupational-related situations that occur during the summer months. Additionally, the reproductive cycles of some snakes are limited by seasons, with egg laying and hatching in the summer. For 1 study, this coincided with the main peaks in people being bitten by snakes, with most incidents for 1 type of snake occurring in the hottest peaks of the day.[23]

Snake venoms are very complex substances, as each contains more than 100 different proteins and peptides.[22] The enzymes found in snake venoms include digestive hydrolases, hyaluronidase-spreading factor, and enzymes that are procoagulants. Additionally, some have neurotoxins that cause paralysis by blocking the presynaptic and postsynaptic neuromuscular junctions.[22]

Snake bite management includes moving the victim to the hospital as quickly and as passively as possible. Excitement, fear, and anxiety cause sympathetic nervous system activation, which will enhance the bodily distribution of the venom. Compression should be used for the whole limb, and pressure via the pressure-pad method might be used and has been shown to be effective in a field trial.[24] The application of nitroglycerin cream or ointment might slow the spread of the venom through the lymphatic system when applied to the affected limb.[22,25]

For several species of snakes, antivenom has been shown to be the only effective antidote in reducing mortality, ameliorating coagulopathies, and reversing neurotoxicities.[22] Reactions to the antivenom can occur and should be treated with epinephrine. They are typically reactions of the type 1 sensitivity.

When the patient comes to the intensive care area, any signs of respiratory distress warrant endotracheal intubation and mechanical ventilation. Hypotension or shock should be treated with plasma expanders or inotropes that are vasoconstrictors. Other issues the patient might face are oliguria or acute kidney injury, infection, necrosis, compartment syndrome, and opthalmia.[22] The critical care nurse should be aware that these complications may ensue and should remain vigilant, as these complications can be caused by the snake venom or the antivenom.

Table 2
Bites and stings more likely to occur in the summer

Name	Source of Bite or Sting	Signs and Symptoms	Venom Content
Cnidarians Jellyfish, Coelenterates, Portuguese-man-o'-war	Discharge from tentacles Tentacles are abundant, with millions of stinging capsules	Urticaria like burning and swelling to affected area Fever, dyspnea, and muscle weakness with extensive exposure or in small children. The box jellyfish (*Chironex fleckeri*) have caused some fatalities in the Pacific regions, as Portuguese- man-o'-war have also caused fatalities[22]	Active toxic ingredient of some is a venom which is a nondialysable protein The burning pain and urticaria are due to the venom containing 5-hydroxytryptamine Paralysis and edema are the result of tetramine and an unidentified protein[26]
Venomous Lizards Mexican beaded lizards, and gila monsters are only lizards of concern in the United States	Venom from submandibular glands is inoculated by mandibular teeth	Bite only when provoke and cling tenaciously causing pain and swelling that radiates Additionally, dizziness, weakness, nausea, vomiting, diaphoresis, dyspnea, hypotension, tachycardia, and angioedema may occur Signs accompanied by neutrophil leukocytosis, thrombocytopenia, mild coagulopathy, and EKG changes[22]	This venom contains tissue-kallikrein-like enzyme releasing bradykins and several peptides including exendin-4
Venomous Fish Stingrays and scorpionfish in the United States Weeverfish in the United Kingdom Stonefish in Asia	Venom glands located in grooves of the spines or beneath a membrane covering the precaudal spine of the stingray	Immediate excruciating pain that is tender, hot, accompanied by erythematous swelling that spreads Infections can be the result of bacteria in the remaining spines of the ray Lacerations can occur with larger fish Other than weeverfish bites, nausea, vomiting, respiratory distress, neurologic impairment, and convulsions can occur[22]	Stingray and weeverfish venoms contain enzymes, thermolabile peptides, and vasoactive compounds such as histamines, catecholamines, and kinins, as well as 5-hydroxytryptamine[22]
Scorpions United States: *Centruroides* *Exilicauda*, Mexico: *Centruroides* species	Scorpions do not bite; they sting The anatomical part that contains the stinger is called a telson The telson is the rearmost segment of the scorpion's body	Initially, Intense pain with rapidly subsequent systemic reactions such as vomiting, diaphoresis, piloerection, variant bradycardia to tachycardia, diarrhea, and priapism Later symptoms include hypertension, shock, pulmonary edema, EKG changes, muscle spasms, dysphagia, hemolysis, acute kidney injury, and thrombotic strokes[22]	Venoms in scorpions include endogenous acetylcholine and catecholamines, which produce initial cholinergic symptoms then later adrenergic symptoms[22]

Abbreviation: EKG, electrocardiogram.

SPIDERS

Most spiders are venomous, but only a few species are actually dangerous to people. Although spider bites are very common in some parts of the world, fatalities associated with spider bites are few.[22] In the south and south central United States, the *Loxosceles recluse*, more commonly known as the brown recluse spider, was the cause of at least 6 deaths in the last century. Fatalities have been reported in the United States and Australia from the *Loxosceles mactans*, as well.[22]

Loxosceles spiders have been shown to cause necrotic systemic spider bite poisoning. Bites usually occur when the victim is sleeping or dressing, and are usually initially painless and unnoticed. As such, these commonly occur indoors, and unlike the other bites under discussion, are not necessarily more common during summer months. Over several hours, a burning sensation occurs at the site of bite, with edema and a macular lesion. A blackened area of eschar develops and typically sloughs off in a few weeks, leaving a necrotic ulcer. About 10% of these bites bring about systemic symptoms such as fever, malaise, headaches, rash, jaundice, hemoglobinemia, and intravascular hemolysis. Acute kidney injury may result, and the rate of fatalities for these bites is about 5%.[22]

OTHER BITES AND STINGS

Summer months are laden with outdoor activities, not only for people, but for many species of animals that have the potential to bite and sting. The first line of defense is prevention. Knowing basic habits and conditions related to one's cohabitation with biting and stinging animals is essential. **Table 2** provides an overview of some of the animals that bite and sting that might be encountered during the summer months, during outdoor activities.

SUMMARY

Bite and sting injuries from dogs, cats, insects, and spiders can initially appear to be benign and uncomplicated, yet they can lead to some devastating conditions for the victim. Infections, pain, disfigurement, tissue damage, allergic reactions, disease, and even mortality can be the result of these bites. Mosquitoes and tick bites are associated with potentially debilitating and life-threatening diseases such West Nile virus, and Lyme disease.[15] Caring for these patients in the critical care setting can be challenging due to the rarity of having these patients admitted to the hospital, and the seasonal nature of bites and stings.

REFERENCES

1. Sacks R, Kerr K. Clinical communications: adults: a 42 year old woman with septic shock: an unexpected source. J Emerg Med 2012;42(3):275–8.
2. Steele MT, Ma OJ, Nakase J, et al. Epidemiology of animal exposure presenting to emergency departments. Acad Emerg Med 2007;14(5):398–403.
3. Sacks JJ, Kresnow M, Houston B. Dogbites: how big a problem? Inj Prev 1996;2: 52–4.
4. Centers for Disease Control and Prevention. Dog-bite related fatalities—United States 1995–1996. MMWR Morb Mortal Wkly Rep 1997;46:463–7.
5. Ambro BT, Wright RJ, Heffelfinger RN. Management of bite wounds in the head and neck. Facial Plast Surg 2010;26(6):456–63.
6. Goldstein EJ. Bite wound and infection. Clin Infect Dis 1992;14:643–50.

7. Taplitz RA. Managing bite wounds. Currently recommended antibiotics for treatment and prophylaxis. Postgrad Med 2004;116:49–52, 55–56, 59.
8. Stierman KL, Lloyd KM, De Luca-Pytell DM, et al. Treatment and outcome of human bites in the head and neck. Otolaryngol Head Neck Surg 2003;128:795–801.
9. Centers for Disease Control and Prevention. Rabies in the US and around the world. Available at: http://www.cdc.gov/rabies/location/index.html. Accessed February 22, 2013.
10. Nguyen D. Epidemiology of animal bites among military personnel in central Germany. Mil Med 1988;153:307–8.
11. Sinclair LL, Zhou C. Descriptive epidemiology of animal bites in Indiana, 1990–1992—rationale for intervention. Public Health Rep 1995;110:64–7.
12. Matter HC. The epidemiology of bite and scratch injuries in vertebrate animals in Switzerland. Eur J Epidemiol 1998;14:483–90.
13. Stefanopoulos PK, Tarantzopoulou AD. Management of facial wound bites. Dent Clin North Am 2009;53:691–705.
14. Holst E, Rollof J, Larsson L, et al. Characterization and distribution of *Pasteurella* species recovered from infected humans. J Clin Microbiol 1992;30:2984–7.
15. O'Neill ME, Mack KA, Gilchrist J. Epidemiology of non-canine bite and sting injuries treated in the US emergency departments, 2001–2004. Public Health Reports 122(2007):764–75.
16. CDC insects and scorpions, NIOSH fast facts. Available at: http://www.cdc.gov/niosh/topics/insects. Accessed February 22, 2013.
17. Tracy JM, Khan FS, Demain JG. Insect anaphylaxis: where are we? The stinging facts 2012. Curr Opin Allergy Clin Immunol 2012;12(4):400–5.
18. Bilo MB. Anaphylaxis caused by *Hymenoptera* stings: from epidemiology to treatment. Allergy 2011;66(Suppl 95):35–7.
19. Kemp SF, Lockey RF, Simons FE. Epinephrine: the drug of choice for anaphylaxis a statement of the World Allergy Organization. Allergy 2008;63:1061–70.
20. Lieberman P, Nicklas RA, Oppenheimer J, et al. The diagnosis and management of anaphylaxis practice parameter: 2011. J Allergy Clin Immunol 2011;126:477–80.
21. Manivannan V, Campbell RL, Bellolio MF, et al. Factors associated with repeated use of epinephrine for treatment of anaphylaxis. Ann Allergy Asthma Immunol 2009;103:395–400.
22. Warrell DA. Venomous bites, stings and poisoning. Infect Dis Clin North Am 2012;26:207–23.
23. Mederios CR, Hess PL, Nicoleti AF, et al. Bites by the colubrid snake *Philodryas patagoniessis*: a clinical and epidemiological study of 297 cases. Toxicon 2010;56:1018–24.
24. Tun-Pe, Aye-Aye-Myint, Khin-Aye-Han, et al. Local compression pads as a first-aid measure for victims of bites by Russell's viper (*Daboia russelii siamensis*) in Myanmar. Trans R Soc Trop Med Hyg 1995;89:293–5.
25. Saul ME, Thomas PA, Dosen PJ, et al. A pharmacological approach to first aid treatment for snakebite. Nat Med 2011;17(7):809–11.
26. Benmeir P, Rosenberg L, Sagi A, et al. Jellyfish envenomation: a summer epidemic. Burns 1990;16(6):471–2.

Bee and Wasp Stings
Reactions and Anaphylaxis

Benjamin A. Smallheer, PhD, RN, ACNP-BC, CCRN[a,b,*]

KEYWORDS

- Bee sting • Wasp sting • Hymenoptera • Anaphylaxis • Reaction
- Venom-specific immunotherapy • Epinephrine

KEY POINTS

- Anaphylaxis involves the integumentary, respiratory, cardiovascular, or gastrointestinal organ systems.
- Anaphylaxis involves 1 organ system no more than 4 hours between the sting and onset of symptoms or 2 or more organ systems no more than 4 hours after the sting whether treated or untreated.
- Vespid venom contains similar allergens creating a high degree of cross-reactivity between insects within this group.
- Hymenoptera venom hypersensitivity is the second most prevalent cause of systemic allergic reactions, behind drug-induced systemic allergic reactions.
- Individuals who experience heavy exposure to bees and wasps are at increased likelihood of developing systemic allergic reactions to stings.
- Bees feed on pollen and nectar, whereas wasps have a carnivorous nature.
- Bees have a barbed stinger, which becomes lodged in its victim, typically allowing a single sting.
- Wasps lack barbs on their stinger, allowing them to sting their prey repeatedly.
- Symptoms of an allergic reaction develop within minutes.
- Anaphylactic reactions can be fatal within 30 minutes.
- Reactions may be cutaneous, large local, biphasic, or systemic in nature.
- Integumentary, gastrointestinal, and immunologic symptoms are the most common physiologic responses to an insect sting.
- Atypical responses to stings may occur in the cardiovascular, genitourinary, gynecologic, hematologic, musculoskeletal, neurologic, ocular, pulmonary, and renal systems.
- Prediction of risk of systemic reaction to future stings is primarily based on the severity of past reactions, history and degree of exposure, age of the patient, and the level of sensitivity measured by either a skin test or radioallergosorbent test.

Continued

Disclosures: None.
[a] Vanderbilt University School of Nursing, 461 21st Avenue South, 305 Godchaux Hall, Nashville, TN 37240, USA; [b] Special Care/Rapid Response Team, St. Thomas Hospital, 4220 Harding Road, Nashville, TN 37205, USA
* 461 21st Avenue South, 305 Godchaux Hall, Nashville, TN 37240, USA.
E-mail address: benjamin.a.smallheer@vanderbilt.edu

Crit Care Nurs Clin N Am 25 (2013) 151–164
http://dx.doi.org/10.1016/j.ccell.2013.02.002
0899-5885/13/$ – see front matter © 2013 Elsevier Inc. All rights reserved.

ccnursing.theclinics.com

Continued

- Venom-specific immunotherapy (VIT) is the standard form of immunotherapy used for sting allergy.
- Improvements in quality of life with VIT compared with epinephrine self-injector alone support the use of VIT not only for physiologic indications but for psychological indications as well.
- Education of allergen avoidance is the primary means of treatment.
- Creation of a written emergency action plan helps to streamline self-medication emergency treatment in the event of a reexposure to a sting.

INTRODUCTION

Allergic reactions to bee and wasp stings have been documented since the era of ancient Egypt. One of the legends surrounding the death of the first king of Egypt, Pharaoh Menes in 2640 BC, states that his death was caused by an anaphylactic reaction to a wasp sting.[1] However, it was not until 1902 that Portier and Richet[1] published the seminal work on the phenomenon of anaphylaxis. While at sea, these investigators were attempting to immunize a dog against the venom from tentacles of the sea anemone. After the second injection of the venom, the dog died within minutes. It was from this encounter that the term anaphylaxis was termed.

Numerous definitions and qualifications exist regarding anaphylaxis. The common thread of all definitions states that anaphylaxis typically involves the integumentary, respiratory, cardiovascular, or gastrointestinal (GI) organ systems. In addition, anaphylaxis may or may not include symptom presentation of hypotension or an IgE-mediated hypersensitivity response affecting multiple organ systems.[1,2] This response, if untreated, can cause severe effects, leading to cardiovascular collapse and death. A more technical definition of anaphylaxis outlines the involvement of 1 organ system no more than 4 hours between the sting and onset of symptoms or 2 or more organ systems no more than 4 hours after the sting whether treated or untreated.[3]

All stinging insects have the ability to induce an anaphylactic reaction in their hosts.[4] This article focuses on the Hymenoptera order of insects, specifically bees and wasps. Hymenoptera is the largest order of insects known, and contains suborders of Apidae (bees) and Vespidae (vespids). Apidae includes *Apis mellifera* (honeybees) and *Bombus* species (bumblebees). The suborder of Vespidae (vespids) consists of *Vespula* species (yellow jackets) and *Polistes fuscatus* (hornets and wasps).[4–6] **Table 1** summarizes these orders and suborders. Hymenoptera, meaning membrane-winged, comprises approximately 100,000 species of bees, wasps, and ants.[7] Most of these insects have poison-gland and stinging mechanisms, which are used for acquiring food or fending off predators.

The venom of Hymenoptera insects contains protein allergens, most of which have enzymatic activity. In addition, the venom contains nonallergenic components such as toxins, vasoactive amine molecules, acetylcholine, and kinins.[4,6,8] The venom of the

Table 1
Class/subclasses of Hymenoptera

Order: Hymenoptera	
Suborder: Apidae (bees)	**Suborder: Vespidae (vespids)**
Apis mellifera (honeybees)	*Vespula* species (yellow jackets)
Bombus species (bumblebees)	*Polistes fuscatus* (hornets and wasps)

honey bee is immunochemically distinct from the other Hymenoptera, making cross-reactivity unlikely. However, vespid venom contains virtually the same allergens between suborder, creating a high degree of cross-reactivity between insects within this group.[6]

The stinging apparatus is located at the tail end of the abdominal segment of the insect and is capable of delivering 50 μg of venom. In the absence of allergic responses, it would take approximately 1500 stings to deliver a quantity of venom deemed to be a lethal dose.[5] It is this venom that is capable of inducing toxic or vaso-active responses within the body of the host.

INCIDENCE

The incidence of Hymenoptera venom hypersensitivity[1] is from 0.05% to 5% of the population.[3,7] This prevalence of reactions is second only to drug-induced ana-phylaxis.[9] There are approximately 400,000 visits per year to emergency departments across the United States as result of anaphylaxis of various origins. The location of the individual, and the type of activity in which they were engaged at the time of the sting, are important in determining the most likely cause of the sting.[5] Of these stings, 40 to 100 Americans die every year as a result of severe systemic reactions to bee, wasp, and ant stings.[2,7,10]

Systemic allergic reactions can occur at any age, often after numerous uneventful stings.[6] A medical history of severe sting reactions has been reported by up to 3% of adults and almost 1% of children. In children, a history of systemic allergic reactions can be found documented in medical records of at least 0.8% of children.[6] There is evidence that most children do outgrow systemic allergic responses to insect stings; however, 1 in 5 individuals stung up to 32 years after the original reaction still show an allergic reaction.[11] In addition, there is a small documented cross-reactivity between bee and wasp stings and plant allergens such as ragweed, banana, melon, or canta-loupe or with carbohydrate determinates.[6,12,13]

Persons at highest risk for allergic reactions are more commonly persons who expe-rience heavy exposure. Beekeepers and their families are at high risk of becoming allergic because of the high rate of contact and risk of being stung during their regular duties. In such a highly exposed population, up to 31% of individuals report large local reactions, whereas 14% to 32% report systemic allergic reactions.[14] Higher inci-dences of systemic allergic reactions are common in countries and areas where expo-sure is greater. Switzerland, for example, has a large beekeeping industry. Having an increased chance of exposure to multiple stings simultaneously or repeated stings within a single season in addition increases the chance of systemic reactions.[6,14]

After the occurrence of a systemic allergic reaction to a sting, the risk of a repeat reaction increases. Sensitization to venom from the sting occurs in more than 30% of adults in the weeks after a sting. However, there is evidence that sensitization may be self-limited in 30% to 50% of cases after 5 to 10 years.[4]

SIMILARITIES BETWEEN BEES AND WASPS

Bees and wasps contain numerous similarities in both appearance and behavior (**Table 2**). These similarities are in part because of bees' evolution from predatory wasps.[15] Externally, both contain an exoskeleton, which minimizes water loss as well as providing protection from predators. Their bodies are divided into 3 regions: head, thorax, and abdomen. The head is the major sensory region of the insect, housing the eyes, antennae, and sensory hairs. Ingestion and partial digestion of food occurs through the head.[8]

Table 2
Similarities and differences between bees and wasps

	Bees	Wasps
Anatomy	Exoskeleton	Exoskeleton
	Visible hair on body	Minimal to no body hair
	Short compact body	Narrow streamline body
	3 body regions:	3 body regions:
	Head	Head
	Contains eyes, antennae, and responsible for sensory and nutrition	Contains eyes, antennae, and responsible for sensory and nutrition
	Thorax	Thorax
	2 pairs of wings	2 pairs of wings
	6 legs	6 legs
	Primary locomotion segment	Primary locomotion segment
	Abdomen	Abdomen
	7 segments	7 segments
	Contains internal organs	Contains internal organs
	Barbed stinger	Nonbarbed stinger
Behavior	Gather pollen and nectar	Minimal pollen transport
	Lay eggs within hive/colony	Carnivorous nature
		Lay eggs within colony or on/in prey
Living	Bees	Yellow jackets
	Live in hives/colonies	Ground-dwelling colonies
	Tree hollows, logs, commercial hives	Social and solitary living species
	Social living	Hornets
	Bumble bees	Large papier-mâché nests
	Protected structures	Social living
	Deserted small rodent nests, dead grass piles, or garden substrate	Wasps
	Social and solitary living species	Paperlike honeycomb nests
		Mud nests
		Social living

The antennae are the noses of the insect and contain a 10-segment flagellum used to smell. Two different types of eyes exist on the insect's head: the ocelli and the compound eye. The ocelli consist of 3 eyes located on the top of the head and are arranged in a triangular pattern. The predominate function of the eyes is to detect light intensity. The compound eyes provide a wide range of photoreceptive functions. Each eye is composed of approximately 6900 hexagonal facets, each of which functions as its own independent structure.[8]

The thorax is made up of 3 segments, each of which bears 1 pair of legs, whereas the posterior 2 thoracic segments have 2 pairs of wings. The wings contain powerful muscles for flight, which make the thorax the primary propulsive region of the body.[8,15]

The abdomen is made up of 7 visible segments. This structure contains most of the internal organ systems, some glands, and the stinger.[8] However, only female bees and wasps can sting, because the stinger is a modified egg-laying structure not present in males.[15]

DIFFERENCE BETWEEN BEES AND WASPS

Evolutionary differences exist between bees and wasps. These differences help distinguish between the 2 within the environment. Bees are visibly hairy, and the fur is distributed across their legs and abdomen for pollen collection. The hairs distributed on their legs are used to clean dust and pollen from the head and thorax and for pollen sac collection.[8] Wasps have no fur and therefore are less able to carry pollen. Any pollen collection while visiting flowers is unintentional. Wasps typically have an elongate body, longer legs, and a very narrow waist, whereas bees are usually more compact. These anatomic differences permit a wasp to fly faster than a bee.[8,15]

Bees are well recognized for their gathering of pollen and nectar from flowers to use as food for their colonies and offspring. Wasps are carnivorous, and although they are attracted by sweet foods, they also hunt other insects as a primary source of food.[5] These insects include common garden pests such as aphids, tomato hornworms, cabbage worms, and strawberry leaf rollers.[15] Wasps often use their hosts as a nutrition source for their young. Whereas bees lay their eggs within the combs of the colony, wasps may lay their eggs within a nest or either on or in their host. This practice allows the larva to feed on the host as it matures into a grown wasp, eventually killing and devouring the host.[15]

However, the greatest difference between bees and wasps is the stinger. Honeybees have a barbed stinger with an attached venom sac. The 2-barbed stinger quickly saws its way into the victim and becomes lodged in the skin of the predator. Because of this mechanism, the stinger typically remains in the victim's flesh after the sting. As the bee pulls away, the venom sac and internal organs are eviscerated from the bee's body, causing death to the bee within hours to days. However, this mechanism allows the stinging apparatus to continue to pump venom into the flesh of the predator for 30 to 60 seconds after evisceration from the bee's body as the muscles surrounding the poison sac contract.[5,8]

Bumblebees' stingers have fewer barbs than a honeybee's stinger, and can therefore sting repeatedly because evisceration is less likely after a single sting. Similar to the bumblebee, wasps, hornets, and yellow jackets lack barbs on their stinger, making them capable of stinging predators or prey numerous consecutive times.[7]

LIVING ENVIRONMENT
Honey Bees

Honeybees live in hives. Domestic honeybees reside in commercial hives and are easily observed on flowers in nature. However, wild honeybees' nests can be found in tree hollows, logs, and even in the sides of buildings. Their hives may contain thousands of docile bees, which can become aggressive around their hives during cool and damp weather or when provoked.[5,7]

Africanized honeybees are an especially aggressive hybrid between domestic honeybees and African honeybees. This hybrid is the result from an experiment intended to enhance honey production. This hybrid breed was accidentally introduced into South America and has been migrating northward over the years. They can now be found in several of the southern states of the United States.[5,6] African honeybees live in colonies and although their venom is no different than that of other honeybees, because of their swarm-and-attack behavior, the number of stings from an encounter is excessive and can therefore be fatal.[6,7]

Bumblebees

Bumblebees are slow moving and nonaggressive. Stings from a bumblebee are rare, unless the insect is provoked. Bumblebees live in colonies in the ground, in commercial hives, protected structures, or even deserted small rodent nests, dead grass piles, or garden substrate.[5,7]

Bumblebees have social and solitary species, which are seasonal in nature. The colonies die out in late autumn and the queens hibernate underground to start a new colony the following year.[15]

Yellow Jackets

Yellow jackets have ground-dwelling colonies, and because of their urbanized nature, are typically encountered by innocent individuals during yard work, gardening, or farming.[5,7] When their nests are disturbed, the yellow jackets become aggressive in an effort to defend their colony. It is for this reason that yellow jacket stings are common and are also the most common cause of sting-induced allergic reactions in most areas.[4] In addition, yellow jackets have been known to follow their predators and sting them repeatedly over distances. Yellow jackets are often found associated with food in the outdoor setting, especially in late summer, when native sources of food begin to get scarce.[5,7,15] It is because of the wasps' attraction to food that stings in the mouth, oropharynx, and esophagus are common.

Yellow jackets, like bumblebees, have social and solitary species. Yellow jackets also have seasonal colonies that die out in late autumn and the queens hibernate underground to start a new colony the following year.[15]

Hornets

Hornets build large papier-mâché nests, which may span several feet in diameter. These nests are usually found in trees or shrubs and use natural protection from the vegetation. Hornets are aggressive when a predator is within the vicinity of the nest, and like yellow jackets, have been known to follow and sting their predator numerous times over distances away from the nest.[5]

Wasps

Wasps build paperlike honeycomb nests or mud nests several inches or more in diameter. These nests are found in shrubs, under eaves of houses or barns, within pipes on playgrounds, or under patio furniture. The variety of locations chosen by the wasps to construct their nests is typically sheltered from direct sun, wind, and rain. These specific locations provide added protection to the nest and young wasps. Wasps are less aggressive than other vespids; however, when the nest is disturbed, they become aggressive and can sting their predators multiple times.[5,7]

VARIED TYPES OF REACTIONS

After a sting by a wasp or bee, the time of onset to a reaction is often rapid. If the individual experiences an anaphylactic reaction, symptoms typically develop within minutes and can be fatal within 30 minutes of the event. Although there is documentation reporting symptom development several hours after an exposure, early treatment is essential for survival.[2,9] Several types of reactions exist, all varying in severity of symptom expression (**Table 3**).

These reactions include:

- Localized/cutaneous reaction
- Large local reaction
- Biphasic reaction
- Systemic reactions (anaphylaxis)

Table 3	
Types of reactions and common symptom expression	
Localized cutaneous	Pain
	Redness
	Swelling
	Pruritus
	Localized area of induration
	Symptoms last several days
Large local reaction	Pain
	Redness
	Swelling
	Pruritus
	Large area of induration often greater than 15 cm
	Symptoms last 10 d
Biphasic reaction	Pain
	Redness
	Swelling
	Pruritus
	Reemergence of symptoms after the appearance of a complete resolution of symptoms
	Symptoms reemerge several hours after initial resolution
Systemic reaction/anaphylaxis	Develops within minutes of sting
	Generalized cutaneous response
	Associated hypotensive shock
	Abdominal or pelvic pain
	Cardiac rhythm disturbances
	Coronary vasospasm
	Angioedema
	Laryngeal edema
	Bronchospasm

Localized/Cutaneous Reactions

Localized cutaneous reactions are the most common of reactions, occurring in 80% of individuals. This type of response is often the sole manifestation in most children. However, adults report 15% localized reactions and often with isolated ancillary symptoms such as hypotension or respiratory complaints.[6,9]

Immediately after a sting, the tissue mounts a localized histamine response to the injected venom. Localized reactions are not IgE mediated, as are systemic reactions, and therefore require only symptomatic treatment rather than systemic treatment.[5] This histamine response causes localized pain, redness, swelling, and pruritus at and around the site of the sting.[3,6,16] This prodrome of symptoms is transient and may persist for up to several days.[1] Localized reactions may also include flushing or allergic rhinoconjunctivitis symptoms. Individuals who experience a more significant localized reaction are at an increased risk of developing a systemic reaction to future stings.[14]

Large Local Reactions

Large localized reactions are characterized by a late-phase IgE-dependent reaction, which typically develops after 12 to 48 hours after the sting. The diameter of the area of induration often exceeds 15 cm and can persist for 5 to 10 days, with a slow dissipation.[4–6,9] The characteristics of a large local reaction include extensive erythema and swelling surrounding the site of the sting, pain, and pruritus.[5]

Biphasic Reaction

Most reactions are uniphasic, meaning from the time of the sting, the symptoms of the reaction, whether localized or systemic, intensify and then gradually subside. These uniphasic reactions respond rapidly to therapy. However, some individuals have a protracted reaction, which is shown as either an incomplete response to treatment or a return of symptoms after an apparent complete resolution of the initial prodrome.[9]

Biphasic reactions have been reported in 1% to 5% of cases after either a bee or wasp sting. Because of this potential reemergence of symptoms, individuals should be observed for 3 to 6 hours after a sting, depending on the severity of the symptoms.[3,6,9]

Systemic Reaction

Systemic reactions, or anaphylaxis, also known as systemic hypersensitivity syndrome,[9] are the most severe of potential allergic responses. The nature of a systemic reaction is caused by an immunologically induced mast cell or basophil mediator release from an IgE-mediated response.[5]

A systemic reaction typically develops within minutes after a sting.[5,14] These reactions are characterized by a generalized cutaneous response with associated hypotensive shock, abdominal or pelvic pain, cardiac rhythm disturbances, coronary vasospasm, laryngeal edema, bronchospasm, or angioedema.[4,5,16] These systemic reactions can become progressively more severe with each sting and show more significant symptoms in a shorter period.[6] For a victim to experience a toxic effect from the venom alone, they must endure a significant number of stings. However, a systemic reaction requires only 1 sting to develop.[5]

PHYSIOLOGIC RESPONSE

Typical physiologic response to an insect sting is a result of histamine and IgE mediator release. These responses include integumentary symptoms, GI symptoms, and immunologic symptoms.

Integumentary Response

The response of the integumentary system is intended to protect the body from the invasion of toxins. Urticaria, erythematous rash, localized swelling, purpuric maculae, flushing, and pruritus are the most common symptoms shown by the skin.[3,9,17] In cases of extensive toxin burden, localized necrosis has been seen.[10] This type of response by the skin warrants medical attention for wound care, debridement, and, based on the severity of the necrotic area, possible skin grafting.

GI Response

The GI system is sensitive to stress and physiologic conditions. After an insect sting, and the associated local or systemic response, the gut shows an abrupt response. Individuals report significant abdominal pain, cramps, and other associated GI symptoms including nausea, diarrhea, and indigestion.[3,6,9,10] These responses by the GI tract are transient, and although discomforting, do not typically cause any long-term effects.

Immunologic Response

The immune response of the body to a sting is complex. In this immunologic mechanism, IgE initially binds to the venom proteins. This binding activates a separate set of receptors known as the high-affinity IgE receptors, located on both mast cells and basophils. This binding causes a release of histamines and other inflammatory mediators, which cause a full body cascade of physiologic changes recognized as symptoms of anaphylaxis:

- Increased bronchial smooth muscle tone
- Vasodilation
- Increase blood vessel permeability
- Myocardial contractility depression[18]

ATYPICAL RESPONSES

Beyond the typical physiologic responses of the body to stings, numerous atypical responses have also been noted. No body system seems to be excluded from the stress response and toxic effects of bee and wasp venom.

Cardiac

Hypotension is a common outcome associated with an anaphylactic reaction as distributive shock sets in. Numerous cases of hypotension, defined as a systolic blood pressure less than 100 mm Hg, have been documented.[2,3,9,10,17] Increased troponin levels in the absence of chest pain indicate the occurrence of silent myocardial infarctions after several wasp stings to the head and arms of individuals.[17] Holosystolic murmurs, bradycardia, arrhythmias, and angina have also been reported.[6,10]

The development of coronary vasospasm and an ensuing myocardial infarction secondary to the allergic reaction have been described since 1991 as the Kounis syndrome.[19] Kounis syndrome is the development of an acute coronary syndrome induced by allergic or hypersensitivity reactions, such as that to stings. Kounis syndrome can be classified as a type I occurrence or a type II occurrence. Type I includes patients with normal coronary anatomy, in whom the allergic response causes either coronary vasospasm, leading to unstable angina with normal cardiac enzymes, or coronary artery spasm, progressing to acute myocardial infarction.[19] A type II response includes patients with preexisting atherosclerotic disease. This history of coronary artery disease may be known or unknown by the patient. The catecholamine surge and stress from the acute allergic episode can lead to plaque rupture, leading to an acute myocardial infarction.[19]

Genitourinary/Gynecology

Although the documented occurrence of genitourinary/gynecology affects from bee and wasp stings are minimal, there is notation in the literature of fetal demise in pregnant women. In these cases, the woman experienced a spontaneous abortion of what appeared to be a normally developing fetus.[6]

Hematologic

By the nature of allergic reactions, the hematologic system is highly involved in this response. It is not surprising that severe, yet atypical hematologic responses may be experienced by individuals who receive stings by bees or wasps. Beyond the anticipated response of swelling, urticaria, and angioedema, documentation exists surrounding the development of serum sickness, vasculitis, hemolysis, and thrombocytopenia purpura.[5,17] The incidence of chronic urticaria and cold urticaria has also been noted to develop after a sting.[6] In more severe reactions and responses, there are noted incidences of coagulation abnormalities, such as disseminated intravascular coagulation and Henoch-Schönlein syndrome.[5,10,17]

Musculoskeletal

Atypical musculoskeletal effects from allergic responses to stings have been documented to include joint swelling and arthralgias.[10] Large-scale muscle damage, presenting itself clinically as rhabdomyolysis, has been noted after hornet stings.[17]

Neurologic

Significant neurologic effects associated with systemic reactions from bee and wasp stings have been documented as well. These effects include acute disseminated encephalomyelitis, Guillain Barré syndrome, myasthenia gravis, other demyelinating diseases, peripheral neuritis, cerebral infarction, encephalitis, and Reye-like syndrome, which have been reported. In most cases, supportive care and steroid therapy over the course of several months have resulted in resolution of the symptoms.[5,17]

Ocular

Ocular responses can be caused by either direct contact with the sting or the systemic allergic response experienced by the body. Direct trauma from the stinger and venom components have caused ocular lesions, corneal ulcerations and deterioration, and cataracts.[17] In addition, conjunctivitis, corneal infiltrates, lens subluxation, lens abscess, and optic neuropathy have been identified in individuals showing allergic responses to stings.[5,17]

Pulmonary

Pulmonary responses, like hematologic responses, are not uncommon. Most individuals experiencing a sting report dyspnea, wheezing, and feelings of airway closure. A potential contributor to such symptoms outside the allergic response and physiologic contributors may be psychological in nature. An individual experiences pain and fear as a result of the sting. These experiences exacerbate feelings of anxiety, leading to vocal cord dysfunction and feelings of dyspnea. However, atypically, diffuse alveolar hemorrhage and pulmonary edema have been described. These findings have been documented with multiple stings as well as after a single sting.[9,17]

Renal

In cases of systemic allergic responses, renal toxic effects have been documented from as few as 1 single sting to as many as 1700 stings. Cases reported include primary renal failure from both domestic as well as Africanized honeybees, interstitial renal edema and tubular destruction, tubulointerstitial nephritis, and acute nebular nephropathy.[17] In addition, nephrotic syndrome has been reported after just 2 stings.[17]

DIAGNOSTIC TESTS

In making a clinical diagnosis of systemic allergies to bee or wasp stings, significant emphasis should be placed on the individual's history of exposure.[4] When gathering a detailed history, information should be gathered pertaining to all previous stings, the time course until a reaction and of the reaction itself, as well as all associated symptoms and treatments provided. Symptoms may be overestimated by the individual because of experienced fear and panic. Perceptions of throat or chest tightness, dyspnea, lightheadedness, nausea, or other constitutional symptoms may all be attributed to the anxiety, fear, or panic of the event. In addition, heat, alcohol, physical exertion, or underlying cardiopulmonary disease may exaggerate symptom presentation. Performing either a serum assay or a skin test in an individual with no history of a systemic allergic reaction to a sting is not useful in determining an individual's potential for systemic allergic reactions.[6]

Criteria essential for diagnosing an individual with insect sting allergy include:

- Clinical history of a systemic reaction
- Positive venom-specific serum IgE antibody
- Positive venom-specific skin IgE antibody[16]

Performing diagnostic testing for sting allergy is indicated in individuals who have had a systemic reaction. In the absence of known history of an allergic response to a sting, allergy testing is not required because of the low probability of anaphylaxis.[6] One percent of individuals with a history of systemic reactions to a sting show a negative skin test or radioallergosorbent test (RAST). Individuals who show a large local reaction to a sting often have significant results to either a venom skin test or RAST sensitivity. However, they show a low risk of anaphylaxis.[4] In such cases, it may be beneficial to consider the administration of an intentional sting challenge: instigation of an intentional sting by the insect of suspicion.[4] This test should always be performed in a medical facility where emergency treatment can be administered.

The prediction of risk to an individual of systemic reaction to future stings, therefore, is primarily based on the severity of past reactions, history and degree of exposure, the level of sensitivity measured by either a skin test or RAST, and the age of the patient.[4] Other means of diagnosing an allergy include the intentional sting challenge mentioned earlier, in vitro basophil flow cytometry-based assay, and in vitro basophil histamine and sulfidoleukotriene release assay.[16]

TREATMENT PLAN

Treatment plans for allergic reactions vary from venom-specific immunotherapy (VIT), home therapies, emergency medical services/hospital systemic treatment, and education/prevention. Hymenoptera venoms were the first standardized allergens on the market. Whole-body extract (WBE) therapy was the standard treatment of prevention of allergic reactions to stings for almost 50 years.[4] This situation was until WBE was shown to be no better than placebo compared with VIT, which was shown to have a 95% effectiveness.[6] Half of all cases of allergic reactions are considered unpreventable because of the individuals' having no previous knowledge of past allergic reactions. Therefore, emergency treatments were not rapidly sought and the individual would not have been eligible for VIT without knowledge of an allergic history.[4] Referral to an allergy specialist is indicated for evaluation of criteria to receive VIT therapy as well as administration of therapy.[2,16] The process of treatment with immunotherapy decreases the T-cell proliferation after allergen stimulation. In addition, decreased secretion of cytokines and interleukins leads to a suppression of the IgE-mediated immune response.[14]

Treatment guidelines support administration of VIT every 4 weeks for the first 18 to 24 months of therapy, followed by administration every 6 weeks from 18 to 24 months. Therapy is then recommended to be continued every 8 weeks either up to a 5-year period or indefinitely.[4,6] VIT in children reduces the frequency of generalized allergic reactions from 17% to 5% and carries the benefit of offering long-term protection from further generalized reactions in 85% to 95% of cases. However, anaphylaxis may occur with VIT administration, so caution must be exercised with administration.[11,20,21] Improvements in quality of life have been reported with VIT compared with a deterioration found when individuals are given only an epinephrine self-injector. These findings support the use of VIT not only for physiologic indications but for psychological indications as well.[4]

VIT is strongly recommended in individuals with positive RAST as well as a history of moderate to severe systemic allergic reactions to bee or wasp stings. In addition, notable respiratory or cardiovascular symptoms after a sting support VIT.[14] Individuals classified as being involved in high-risk activities, such as beekeeping, should successfully tolerate a sting challenge test performed under clinical conditions before returning to their high-risk activities.[14]

Home Treatment Regimens

After a sting, home treatment regimens should be instituted. Whether the reaction experienced by the individual is localized/cutaneous reaction, or a large localized reaction, treatment should begin immediately. Treatments to be instituted should include:

- Ice to the site of the sting
- Nonsteroidal anti-inflammatory drugs: ibuprofen (Motrin)
- Prostaglandin synthesis inhibitors: acetaminophen (Tylenol)
- Histamine 1 (H_1) inhibitors: famotidine (Pepcid)
- H_2 inhibitors: diphenhydramine (Benadryl)
- Topical application of antihistamine or corticosteroid medications for symptom relief

The use of an epinephrine injector is not recommended in patients who show a large localized reaction, cutaneous systemic reactions, or who are receiving venom immunotherapy.[6] Medical attention should always be sought if the effectiveness of home remedies is in question.

Emergency Medical Services/Hospital Systemic Treatment

Individuals with a known history of systemic allergic reactions should not attempt home remedy treatment. Emergency response assistance should be sought immediately and hospital transport made imminent. Individuals with a known history of systemic allergic reactions should maintain an active prescription for subcutaneous epinephrine injector (1:1000). In addition, when an individual anticipates that they may be in a location where a sting is possible, a subcutaneous epinephrine injection cartridge should be carried with them. First responders are trained in the use of subcutaneous epinephrine injector. In addition, oxygen therapy should be instituted.[2,9,14,16]

After the first administration of epinephrine, if symptoms do not resolve, a second injection of epinephrine should be given. Large-bore intravenous access should be established as soon as possible and the use of antihistamines, hydrocortisone, intravenous fluids, and possible vasopressors should be considered, because clinical manifestations of shock may present. Elevating lower extremities to optimize venous return may be beneficial. If respiratory distress and bronchospasms develop, elevation of the head is more appropriate. Corticosteroid use should be immediately used and measures to secure the airway should be instituted.[2,9,14,16]

The combined use of H_1 and H_2 antihistamines is a second-line agent and is more effective in treatment of the cutaneous manifestations of a generalized allergic reaction such as urticaria, mild angioedema, and pruritus. H_1 antagonists should not be given alone and also should not be attempted as primary and sole therapy for a systemic allergic reaction.[9] In addition, individuals on β-blocker medications may be resistant to epinephrine, because of blockade of the receptor sites needed for epinephrine and other catecholamines to have an effect on the body.[6]

Education

Excessive fear of a reexposure greatly impairs an individual's quality of life.[6] Therefore, education of allergen avoidance is the primary means of treatment. In addition, creation of a written emergency action plan helps to streamline self-medication emergency treatment in the event of a reexposure to a sting.[14,16] During the education process, an individual should also be made aware of the indications of VIT treatment as well as when to carry and use an epinephrine injector. These injectors are indicated for individuals with history of anaphylaxis after a sting.[6,9] If the individual is engaged in activities putting them at an increased risk of exposure, such as beekeeping, the individual either needs to stop the activities, or wear protective clothing.[14] Listings of educational resources and guidelines should include:

- Wearing long trousers and shirts when outside
- Avoiding pollinated plants and grassy areas
- Avoiding perfumes, fragrant soaps, and lotions
- Avoiding eating and drinking outdoors and with straws[2]

SUMMARY

There are many similarities and differences between bees and wasps. In addition, allergic reactions to bee and wasp stings manifest themselves in a variety of ways from simple cutaneous reactions, more complex biphasic reactions, to life-threatening systemic anaphylactic reactions. Treatment may range from home therapies using over-the-counter medications or prescription epinephrine self-injectors to treatment by emergency responders and hospitals, including intravenous medications and intravenous fluids. Education and prevention are the most effective means of treatment. Educating individuals with histories of systemic allergic reactions to avoid situations of likely exposure is essential. Developing an emergency action plan for self-medication administration and seeking of medical attention is a necessary lifesaving step. VIT, when indicated, can provide effective, long-standing treatment against systemic allergic reactions, and improve an individual's quality of life.

REFERENCES

1. Sampson HA. Anaphylaxis and emergency treatment. Pediatrics 2003;111:1601–8.
2. Clark S, Camargo CA Jr. Emergency treatment and prevention of insect-sting anaphylaxis. Curr Opin Allergy Clin Immunol 2006;6:279–83.
3. Clark S, Camargo CA. Epidemiology of anaphylaxis. J Allergy Clin Immunol 2007; 27:145–63.
4. Golden DB. Insect sting allergy and venom immunotherapy: a model and a mystery. J Allergy Clin Immunol 2005;3:439–47.
5. Ellis AK, Day JH. Clinical reactivity to insect stings. Curr Opin Allergy Clin Immunol 2005;5:349–54.
6. Golden DB. Insect sting anaphylaxis. Immunol Allergy Clin North Am 2007;27: 261–72.
7. Steen CJ, Janniger CK, Schutzer SE, et al. Insect sting reactions to bees, wasps, and ants. Int J Dermatol 2005;44:91–4.
8. Winston ML. Form and function: honey bee anatomy. In: The biology of the honey bee. Cambridge (MA): Harvard University Press; 1987. p. 13–45.
9. Brown AF. Current management of anaphylaxis. Emergencias 2009;21:213–23.
10. Gawlik R, Rymarczyk B, Rogala B. A rare case of intravascular coagulation after honey bee sting. J Investig Allergol Clin Immunol 2004;14:250–2.

11. Golden DB, Kagey-Sobotka A, Norman PS, et al. Outcomes of allergy to insect stings in children, with and without venom immunotherapy. N Engl J Med 2004; 351:668–74.
12. Hemmer W, Focke M, Kolarich D, et al. Antibody binding to venom carbohydrates is a frequent cause for double positivity to honeybee and yellow jacket venom in patients with sting-insect allergy. J Allergy Clin Immunol 2001;108:1045–52.
13. Aalberse RC, Koshte V, Clemens JG. Immunoglobulin E antibodies that cross-react with vegetable foods, pollen, and Hymenoptera venom. J Allergy Clin Immunol 1981;68:356–64.
14. Müller UR. Bee venom allergy in beekeepers and their family members. Curr Opin Allergy Clin Immunol 2005;5:343–7.
15. Pawelek J, Coville R. Wasps vs. bees. In: Urban bee gardens. Available at: http://nature.berkeley.edu/urbanbeegardens/general_waspsvsbees.html.   Accessed October 10, 2012.
16. Hamilton RG. Diagnostic methods for insect sting allergy. Curr Opin Allergy Clin Immunol 2004;4:297–306.
17. Reisman RE. Unusual reactions to insect stings. Curr Opin Allergy Clin Immunol 2005;5:355–8.
18. Khan BQ, Kemp SF. Pathophysiology of anaphylaxis. Curr Opin Allergy Clin Immunol 2011;11:319–25.
19. Mytas DZ, Stougiannos PN, Zairis MN, et al. Acute anterior myocardial infarction after multiple bee stings. A case of Kounis syndrome. Int J Cardiol 2009;134: e129–31.
20. Galera C, Soohun N, Zankar N, et al. Severe anaphylaxis to bee venom immunotherapy: efficacy of pretreatment and concurrent treatment with omalizumab. J Investig Allergol Clin Immunol 2009;19:225–9.
21. Brown SG. Clinical features and severity grading of anaphylaxis. J Allergy Clin Immunol 2004;2:371–6.

Tick Bites and Lyme Disease
The Need for Timely Treatment

Maria L. Overstreet, PhD, RN

KEYWORDS

- Tick • Lyme • Vector-borne • Bite • Bacterium

KEY POINTS

- Lyme disease can be prevented with early detection of tick attachment, removal, and treatment.
- Treatment of choice is doxycycline (100 mg twice daily, 10–21 days, orally).
- Prevention includes teaching about the life cycle of ticks, how ticks detect a host, transmission of bacteria, proper removal, when to seek treatment, and necessity of time.

INTRODUCTION

The 6th most common nationally notifiable disease in the United States in 2011 was Lyme disease, also identified as the most reported vector-borne illness.[1] In the United States, 30,158 people were reported as having contracted Lyme disease during 2010.[1] Over an 8-year period (2003–2010), the average number of persons contracting Lyme disease was 26,947 (**Fig. 1**).[2] The initial diagnosis of Lyme disease occurred after an outbreak of arthralgias in a group of pediatric patients in 1977 in and around Lyme, Connecticut. Today, Lyme disease remains a public health concern in 2 main portions of the United States, the northeast and north-central states; 96% of the cases in 2011 were reported from the following 13 states: Connecticut, Delaware, Maine, Maryland, Massachusetts, Minnesota, New Hampshire, New Jersey, New York, Pennsylvania, Vermont, Virginia, and Wisconsin.[1]

Fig. 1 shows the incidence of reported cases of Lyme disease over an 8-year period in the United States.

NATURE OF PROBLEM

Tick bites are considered a vector-borne disease. Bacterium the tick can transmit while attached may result in disease. The bacterium is transmitted to humans by ticks.

Vanderbilt University School of Nursing, Godchaux Hall 603A, 461 21st Avenue South, Nashville, TN 37240, USA
E-mail address: maria.overstreet@vanderbilt.edu

Crit Care Nurs Clin N Am 25 (2013) 165–172
http://dx.doi.org/10.1016/j.ccell.2013.02.013
0899-5885/13/$ – see front matter © 2013 Elsevier Inc. All rights reserved.

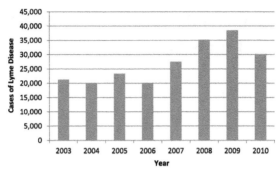

Fig. 1. Cases of Lyme disease in the United States by year. (*Data from* Centers for Disease Control and Prevention. Morbidity and Mortality Weekly Report. Available at: http://www.cdc.gov/mmwr/preview/mmwrhtml/mm5953a1html. Accessed February 21, 2013.)

There are typical times during the life cycle of the tick when the probability of infectious bacterium pathogen transference is higher; thus, it is important to consider the life cycle of the tick. The tick life cycle involves 3 stages: larva, nymph, and adult (**Fig. 2**). During any of these stages, the tick can become infected with bacterium and may transmit bacterium to humans. Approximately 90% of contracted cases are transmitted during the nymph stage of the tick life cycle.[3,4] The nymph's virulence results primarily from the length of time attached to the host: mammals, birds, reptiles, and amphibians are all sources of blood for ticks.[4] A nymph is approximately 2 mm in diameter; therefore, a person may not be aware of a tick's attachment, and the tick may be allowed to feed for an extended period. Time of attachment has become a critical factor in several aspects of Lyme disease. Prolonged attachment allows time for bacterium to move from tick to human.[3,5,6] If a tick is infected, the chance of transmission increases with time attached: 12% at 48 hours, 79% at 72 hours, and 94% at 96 hours of attachment.[7]

SYMPTOMS AND STAGES OF LYME DISEASE

Typically, symptoms of Lyme disease present in 1 of 3 stages (**Fig. 3**). Patients may experience some or all of the symptoms in each stage and may fluctuate in and out

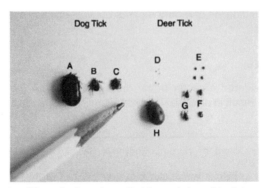

Fig. 2. Tick size during life cycle. Dog (wood) ticks and deer (black-legged) ticks compared with a pencil. Dog ticks: A, engorged female; B, female; and C, male. Deer ticks: D, larvae; E, nymphs; F, males; G, females; and H, engorged female.

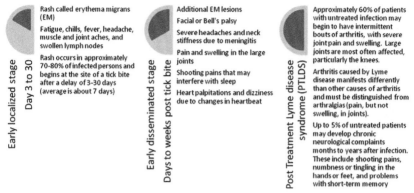

Early localized stage	Day 3 to 30	Rash called erythema migrans (EM)

Fatigue, chills, fever, headache, muscle and joint aches, and swollen lymph nodes

Rash occurs in approximately 70-80% of infected persons and begins at the site of a tick bite after a delay of 3-30 days (average is about 7 days) | |
| Early disseminated stage | Days to weeks post tick bite | Additional EM lesions

Facial or Bell's palsy

Severe headaches and neck stiffness due to meningitis

Pain and swelling in the large joints

Shooting pains that may interfere with sleep

Heart palpitations and dizziness due to changes in heartbeat | |
| Post Treatment Lyme disease syndrome (PTLDS) | | Approximately 60% of patients with untreated infection may begin to have intermittent bouts of arthritis, with severe joint pain and swelling. Large joints are most often affected, particularly the knees.

Arthritis caused by Lyme disease manifests differently than other causes of arthritis and must be distinguished from arthralgias (pain, but not swelling, in joints).

Up to 5% of untreated patients may develop chronic neurological complaints months to years after infection. These include shooting pains, numbness or tingling in the hands or feet, and problems with short-term memory | |

Fig. 3. Signs and symptoms in stages of Lyme disease. (*From* Centers for Disease Control and Prevention. Signs and symptoms of Lyme disease. Available at: http://www.cdc.gov/lyme/signs_symptoms/index.html. Accessed February 16, 2013.)

of each stage. Stage 1, early localized disease, usually occurs a few days to 1 month after a tick bite. The hallmark symptom is erythema migrans, a bull's-eye rash (**Fig. 4**). Nonspecific complaints resemble a viral syndrome, including malaise, fatigue, headache, myalgia, arthralgias, or generalized lymphadenopathy.[3,8] During the period from 1992 through 2004, of the patients reported to have Lyme disease, 68% had erythema migrans, 33% had arthritis, and 1% experienced the severe symptoms of meningitis and heart block.[8]

Stage 2, early disseminated disease, can occur days to 10 months after a tick bite. At this time, symptoms can include those listed for stage 1 in addition to multiple organ involvement, including atrioventricular block, pericarditis, meningeal irritation, and meningitis. Additional symptoms may include palpitations, syncope, dyspnea, stiff neck, photophobia, poor memory, difficulty concentrating, parasthesia and persistent malaise, fatigue, fever, chills, and nausea.[3,7,9] Additional erythema migrans may appear on other parts of the body, possibly resultant from other tick attachments that were not identified.

Stage 3, late persistent disease, late disseminated disease, or chronic Lyme disease, now referred to as *post-treatment Lyme disease syndrome*, may occur months to years after a single tick bite. Patients may present with musculoskeletal and neurologic symptoms, such as arthritis with swelling joints, stiffness, and pain along with

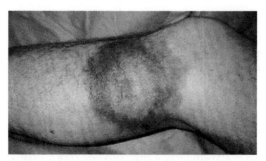

Fig. 4. Erythema migrans. (*From* Lewis S, Dirksen SR, Heitkemper MM. Medical surgical nursing: assessment and management of clinical outcomes. St Louis (MO): Mosby; 2011. p. 1662; with permission.)

myalgia, fatigue, ataxia, mood changes, sleep disturbances, and personality changes.[3,7,9]

Patients in critical care with Lyme disease left untreated may result in varying degrees of permanent damage. Chances of recovery are based on the early recognition of symptoms and treatment. Treatment of chronic Lyme disease may elicit full recovery, or patients may be left with any or all of the symptoms listed in **Table 1**.[7,10] Approximately 10% to 20% of patients with confirmed Lyme disease may have symptoms that last months to years after treatment.[10] Post-treatment Lyme disease syndrome is thought to be due to the body's autoimmune response: the body continues to elicit an autoimmune response when no longer needed, thus causing further damage to the body's tissues.

PHYSIOLOGY OF LYME DISEASE

It is postulated the immune system plays an integral role in the development of the various stages of Lyme disease. The body's inability to mount a sufficient immune response may be responsible for the severity of the initial or late stages of this disease.

Tick saliva also may play a role in the survival of the bacterium.[11] Within the saliva, a protein may suppress the local immunoreactivity, allowing the bacterium to enter a person and spread more quickly. It is also postulated that specific binding properties may allow the bacterium to disseminate more quickly to certain target tissues, such as the central nervous system.[11] Some investigators postulate that problems may exist in the regulation of the trafficking and activation of the inflammatory cells. Hu[11] states Borrelia burgdorferi does not produce destructive molecules or toxins, thus the majority of symptoms are subject to the host immune response.

Coinfection is thought to influence a host's defense mechanisms adversely.[12] Researchers from the National Institute of Allergy and Infectious Diseases have demonstrated mice coinfected with human granulocytic ehrlichiosis, now referred to as *human granulocytic anaplasmosis*, suffered increased severity of Lyme disease.[12] Human granulocytic anaplasmosis and babesiosis may be found as coinfectious agents in patients who have Lyme disease.[7,13–15]

DIAGNOSIS OF LYME DISEASE

A thorough patient history and a meticulous skin inspection are the 2 most important elements used for the diagnosis of Lyme disease. Patient report of symptoms and the

Table 1	
Symptoms of untreated Lyme disease	
Body System	**Symptoms of Untreated Lyme Disease**
Musculoskeletal system	Joints with pain and swelling progressing to arthritis
Central nervous system	Facial nerve paralysis, visual disturbances, meningitis, encephalitis, memory loss, difficulty concentrating, mood changes, personality changes, and altered sleeping habits
Cardiac system	Irregularities of heart rhythm, carditis, and transient atrioventricular blocks of varying degree

Data from Massachusetts Department of Public Health, Division of Epidemiology and Immunization. Tickborne diseases in Massachusetts: a physician's reference manual. 2nd edition. Available at: http://www.mass.gov/eohhs/docs/dph/cdc/lyme/tickborne-diseases-physician-manual.pdf. Accessed February 20, 2013, with permission; and *From* Marques A. Chronic Lyme disease: a review. Infect Dis Clin North Am 2008;22:341–60; with permission.

occurrence of and exposure to ticks in endemic areas may be the only clues to the cause of a patient's current symptoms. Diagnosis of infection remains controversial: some researchers maintain that a diagnosis of Lyme disease can be made on clinical grounds with serologies considered solely in a supportive role.[16,17] Blood tests may confirm Lyme disease, but a negative blood test accompanied with positive symptomology, typically including erythema migrans, is considered positive for Lyme disease.[16]

Laboratory Tests

Blood tests for Lyme disease measure the body's production of antibodies to *Borrelia burgdorferi*. These tests are not able to detect acute infection until the body has been able to produce measurable amounts of antibodies, sometimes not until 2 to 8 weeks after the bite. The Centers for Disease Control and Prevention currently recommend a 2-tier test for Lyme disease. The first test is an enzyme immunoassay (EIA).[18] If the EIA is negative, no further testing is recommended. If the EIA is positive or indeterminate, a second-tier test is then performed. The second-tier test is an immunoblot test, commonly called *Western blot*. Positive results from EIA and Western blot are considered indicative of Lyme disease. These results can take time, and treatment should be initiated with a positive patient history and symptoms without waiting for test results.[16]

Caution

Some laboratories have begun to market and offer tests for the diagnosis of Lyme disease and have not received approval from the Food and Drug Administration as accurate tests for Lyme disease. Without adequately establishing accuracy for the tests, the approved clinical usefulness is questioned (see the Centers for Disease Control and Prevention Web site for a listing of these unapproved tests).[18]

TREATMENT OF LYME DISEASE
Tick Removal

Ticks must be removed promptly to reduce the length of exposure. Patients admitted to a critical care unit with symptoms mimicking Lyme disease must be inspected thoroughly for ticks. Ticks should be removed with precision, using a slow, gentle, pulling motion with disposable tweezers placed as close as possible to a tick's attachment to the skin (**Fig. 5**).[19] After tick removal, the skin should be cleaned to remove any

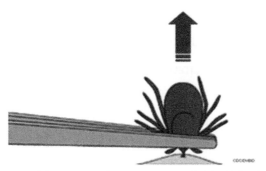

Fig. 5. Proper tick removal demonstrated: use tweezers to hold tick firmly and apply a slow, steady pull for proper removal. (*From* the Centers for Disease Control and Prevention. Tick removal. Available at: http://www.cdc.gov/lyme/removal/index.html. Accessed February 20, 2013.)

bacteria at the site of attachment. The tick should not be touched, because blood and bacteria can be transmitted to the nurse. Good hand-washing practices must be used. It is important to document where the tick was attached and any signs of a rash at the site of attachment. A rash can appear up to 1 month after removal; therefore, follow-up with a primary health care provider is encouraged.

Antibiotics

Lyme disease can be treated effectively with antibiotic therapy, but routine prophylactic use of antimicrobials is not recommended.[13] Some experts recommend antibiotic therapy only if certain symptoms appear or if specific epidemiologic information is available (eg, the accurate determination of the species of tick and degree of engorgement). These data, however, are not routinely available. The most common drug of choice is doxycycline. Doxycycline (100 mg taken orally twice daily for 10 to 21 days) is typical treatment of both stage 1 and stage 2 Lyme disease.[7,13,20,21] Cefuroxime axetil or erythromycin can be used (particularly in pregnant women) if patients are allergic to penicillin or cannot take tetracyclines.[20] Treatment of third-stage, or chronic, Lyme disease may involve vigorous intravenous antibiotic therapy as well as continued investigation for other possible causes.

PREVENTION OF LYME DISEASE

Preventative measures and early recognition of symptoms are keys to inhibiting the occurrence of later stages of Lyme disease. Patients should be taught how to avoid future tick exposure using personal and environmental means of prevention. Ticks find their hosts by several senses: odor, moisture, heat, and vibration.[6] Avoidance of tick-infested areas, such as wooded areas or leaf piles, is paramount. Patients who enjoy hiking should stay near the center of paths, routinely perform thorough naked-body inspection, and remove ticks promptly. Tick repellents should be applied while hikers are in wooded areas but should be washed off immediately afterward. Washing with a cloth provides enough gentle friction to disturb a tick's connection to skin if performed immediately after attachment.

SUMMARY

Lyme disease can be prevented with early detection of tick attachment, removal, and treatment. Doxycycline (100 mg twice daily, orally) is the treatment of choice. Prevention includes teaching about the life cycle of ticks, how ticks detect a host, transmission of bacteria, proper removal, when to seek treatment, and necessity of time. Caution is issued with the use of laboratory tests for the diagnosis of Lyme disease from laboratories not approved by the Food and Drug Administration.

WEB SITES OF INTEREST NOT CITED IN THE ARTICLE

American Lyme Disease Foundation http://www.aldf.com
Lyme Disease Foundation http://www.lyme.org
National Institute of Arthritis and Musculoskeletal and Skin Diseases. National Institutes of Health http://www.niams.nih.gov.

REFERENCES

1. Centers for Disease Control and Prevention. Statistics on Lyme disease. Available at: http://www.cdc.gov/lyme/stats/index.html. Accessed February 16, 2013.

2. Centers for Disease Control and Prevention. Morbidity and Mortality Weekly Report. Available at: http://www.cdc.gov/mmwr/preview/mmwrhtml/mm5953a1 html. Accessed February 21, 2013.
3. Sigal LH. Epidemiology and clinical manifestations of Lyme disease. Up to date. Available at: http://www.uptodateonline.com/application/topic/print.asp?file=othr _inf/6836&;type=A&s. Accessed February 20, 2013.
4. Centers for Disease Control and Prevention. Lifecycle of blacklegged ticks. Available at: http://www.cdc.gov/lyme/transmission/blacklegged.html/. Accessed February 20, 2013.
5. Sigal LH. Bacteriology and epidemiology of Lyme disease. Up to date. Available at: http://www.uptodateonline.com/utd/content/topic.do?topicKey=tickflea/7074 &;view=print. Accessed February 20, 2013.
6. Centers for Disease Control and Prevention. Life cycle of hard ticks that spread disease. Available at: http://www.cdc.gov/ticks/life_cycle_and_hosts.html. Accessed February 20, 2013.
7. Massachusetts Department of Public Health, Division of Epidemiology and Immunization. Tickborne diseases in Massachusetts: a physician's reference manual. 2nd edition. Available at: http://www.mass.gov/eohhs/docs/dph/cdc/lyme/tick borne-diseases-physician-manual.pdf. Accessed February 20, 2013.
8. Centers for Disease Control and Prevention. Reported clinical findings among Lyme disease patients. Available at: http://www.cdc.gov/ncidod/dvbid/lyme/ld_ bysymptoms.htm. Accessed February 20, 2013.
9. Centers for Disease Control and Prevention. Signs and symptoms of Lyme disease. Available at: http://www.cdc.gov/lyme/signs_symptoms/index.html. Accessed February 16, 2013.
10. Marques A. Chronic lyme disease: a review. Infect Dis Clin North Am 2008;22: 341–60.
11. Hu L. Immunopathogenesis of Lyme Disease. Up to date. Available at: http://www.uptodate.com.proxy.library.vanderbilt.edu/contents/immunopathogenesis-of-lyme-disease?source=search_result&search=Lyme+disease&selectedTitle=10% 7E150. Accessed March 23, 2013.
12. National Institute of Allergy and Infectious Diseases. National Institutes of Health. NIAID Research. Co-infection. Available at: http://www.nih.gov/research/topics/ lyme/research/co-infection/. Accessed February 20, 2013.
13. Wormser GP, Nadelman RJ, Dattwyler RJ, et al. Practice guidelines for the treatment of Lyme disease. Clin Infect Dis 2000;31(Suppl 1):S1–14.
14. White DJ, Talarico J, Chang HG, et al. Human babesiosis in New York State: review of 139 hospitalized cases and analysis of prognostic factors. Arch Intern Med 1998;158:212149–54.
15. Bakken JS, Krueth J, Wilson-Nordskog C, et al. Clinical and laboratory characteristics of human granulocytic ehrlichiosis. JAMA 1996;275:199–205.
16. Bransfield PS, Sherr V, Smith H, et al. Evaluation of antibiotic treatment in patients with persistent symptoms of Lyme disease: an ILADS position paper. Bethesda (MD): The International Lyme and Associated Diseases Society; 2003.
17. Centers for Disease Control and Prevention. Lyme disease diagnosis. Available at: http://www.cdc.gov/ncidod/dvbid/lyme/ld_humandisease_diagnosis.htm. Accessed February 20, 2013.
18. Centers for Disease Control and Prevention. Other types of laboratory testing. Available at: http://www.cdc.gov/lyme/diagnosistesting/LabTest/OtherLab/index. html. Accessed February 20, 2013.

19. Centers for Disease Control and Prevention. Tick removal. Available at: http://www.cdc.gov/lyme/removal/index.html. Accessed February 20, 2013.
20. Gilbert DN, Moellering RC, Eliopoulos GM, et al. The Sanford guide to antimicrobial therapy. 36th edition. Hyde Park (VT): Merck; 2006.
21. Stupica D, Lusa L, Ruzić-Sabljić E, et al. Treatment of erythema migrans with doxycycline for 10 days versus 15 days. Clin Infect Dis 2012;55:343–50.

North American Snake and Scorpion Envenomations

Jennifer Wilbeck, DNP, APRN, CEN[a],*, Chip Gresham, MD, FACEM[b]

KEYWORDS

- Snakebite • Rattlesnake • Coral snakes • Scorpion • Envenomations • Antivenom

KEY POINTS

- Among venomous North American snakes and scorpions, the greatest morbidity and mortality is attributable to the effects of the crotalinae family (pit viper), specifically the rattlesnake.
- Antivenom use in North America has historically been most frequently used for rattlesnake envenomations. Although no commercially available coral snake antivenom is currently being produced in the United States, scorpion-specific antivenom was recently approved by the Food and Drug Administration.
- Complications, such as coagulopathies, neurotoxicity, rhabdomyolysis, and, very rarely, compartment syndrome, may occur following snake bites and require holistic, intensive nursing care.
- To optimize patient outcomes, medical toxicologists should be consulted early in the care of patients (via regional poison centers) following snake and scorpion envenomations to assist with procurement of antivenom and identify its appropriate use.

Envenomations by snakes and scorpions in North America, although uncommon, do occur, and the victims may seek medical treatment. Combined, snake and scorpion encounters result in more than 25,000 calls a year to poison centers. Regardless of geographic practice area, exposures will occur that may result in a significant envenomation. The goal of this article was to provide critical care nurses with a fundamental knowledge of varied snake and scorpion envenomation presentations and treatments to assist in optimizing patient outcomes.

SNAKE ENVENOMATIONS
Epidemiology

Although the exact incidence of venomous snake bites is unknown, estimates from the American Association of Poison Control Centers (AAPCC) indicate that nearly 8000

[a] Vanderbilt University School of Nursing, 8228 Donaway Court Brentwood, Nashville, TN 37027, USA; [b] Department of Emergency Medicine, Middlemore Hospital, Auckland, New Zealand
* Corresponding author. 461 21st Avenue South, Nashville, TN 37240, USA.
E-mail address: Jennifer.wilbeck@vanderbilt.edu

Crit Care Nurs Clin N Am 25 (2013) 173–190
http://dx.doi.org/10.1016/j.ccell.2013.02.007
0899-5885/13/$ – see front matter © 2013 Elsevier Inc. All rights reserved.
ccnursing.theclinics.com

individuals sustain venomous snake bites yearly in the United States. Of these bites, fewer than 10 deaths occur annually.[1,2] Estimates from Mexico report up to 27,000 bites annually, resulting in roughly 100 fatalities from rattlesnakes alone.[3] Largely because of the colder climate, numbers of snakebites in Canada are significantly lower, and often result from snakes in private collections. The incidence of snake bites among other countries is not as clearly defined, but worldwide statistics reveal significantly higher numbers of envenomations, as well as greater morbidity and mortality.

Similar to traumatic injuries, snake bites occur more commonly in young adult men, although school-aged children represent a significant percentage of bites as well. The incidence of bites increases among snake handlers and collectors and with use of ethanol or other intoxicants. Additionally, warmer months when snakes, as well as humans, are likely to be more active results in increased environmental encounters and bites.[4,5]

Native venomous snakes have been identified in all states except Alaska, Hawaii, and Maine, with the highest numbers found in the Appalachian, southern, and western areas, and with lower numbers among the New England and northern states. The areas of highest incidence for snakebites are indicated in **Fig. 1**, although venomous snakebite calls have been received from all states except Hawaii.[4] Given this, health care providers throughout North America should maintain a fundamental familiarity with the presentation and management for each of these envenomations.

Although roughly 2500 known species of venomous snakes exist worldwide, approximately 30 species are known to exist in North America. The Viperidae and Elapidae families represent the venomous species of medical importance. Common Viperidae species belong to the subfamily Crotalinae, and include different types of rattlesnakes (*Crotalus* and *Sistrurus* genera), copperheads, and water moccasins (genus *Agkistrodon*). Of the venomous snakebites reported in North America, almost exclusively they are attributable to Crotalinae, or pit vipers. The Elapidae family, including coral snakes, are responsible for the few remaining venomous snake bites.[4,5]

CHARACTERISTICS OF VENOMOUS NORTH AMERICAN SNAKES

Crotalinae and Elapidae snakes each possess distinct characteristics that may aid in identification (**Figs. 2 and 3**). Crotalinae possess a triangular-shaped head with vertically elliptical eyes and a single pair of hollow front fangs. Because of heat-sensing organs, which appear as pitlike depressions in the skin behind their nostrils, snakes in the Crotalinae subfamily are often referred to as "pit vipers." In addition to these general characteristics, specific species of pit vipers demonstrate individually identifying characteristics. Depending on their maturity, rattlesnakes, as their name suggests, may have rattles on their tails that they use as a warning and are often reported to be heard before a strike. Water moccasins, also referred to as "cottonmouths," have a distinct white mouth. Copperheads are reddish-brown in color with hourglass markings on their bodies.

The coral snakes of the Elapidae family in North America are classically known for their brightly colored alternating bands of red, yellow, and black. Because of similar color markings, nonpoisonous king snakes may be easily confused with the coral snake. These 2 snakes can be differentiated by head color and sequencing of the color bands: coral snakes have black snouts, and king snakes have red snouts. In the coral snake, the red and yellow bands are next to each other, but in the king snake, a black band separates the 2 colors. A familiar folk saying may help to recall the differences: "Red on yellow kills a fellow; red on black, venom lack" (see **Fig. 3**).

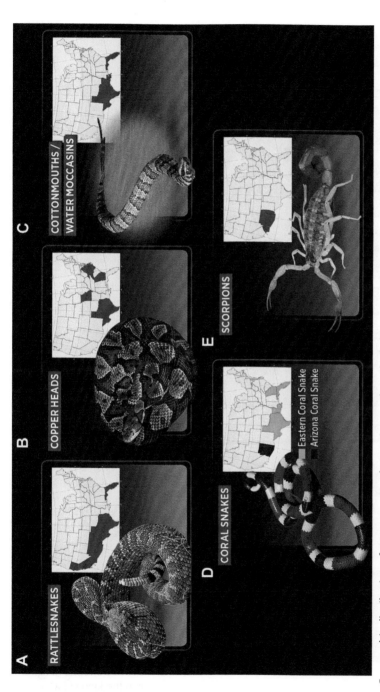

Fig. 1. Geographic distribution of venomous North American snakes. Shaded areas represent states with highest reported bites. Does not include all areas where species have been identified. (*Data from* Bronstein AC, Spyker DA, Cantilena LR, et al. 2011 Annual Report of the American Association of Poison Control Centers' National Poison Data System (NPDS): 29th Annual Report. Clin Toxicol (Phila) 2012;50:911–1164; and *From* [A] Photo credit: Gary Stolz/USFWS; [B] Photo credit: CDC/ Edward J. Wozniak D.V.M., Ph.D.; [C] Photo credit: Pete Pattavina/USFWS; [D] Photo credit: Jeff Servoss/USFWS; and [E] Photo credit: Brian Basgen, Sahuarita, AZ.)

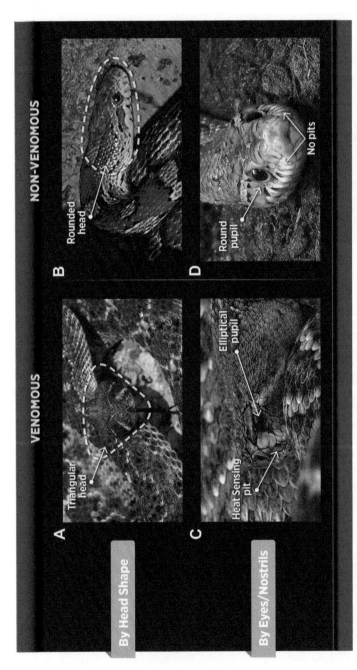

Fig. 2. Identifying features of venomous versus nonvenomous snakes. (*From* [A] Photo credit: Clinton & Charles Robertson, Del Rio, Texas & College Station, TX; [B] Photo credit: " © Patrick JEAN/muséum d'histoire naturelle de Nantes; [C] Photo credit: Joxerra Aihartza; and [D] Photo credit: Linda Tanner, Los Osos, CA.)

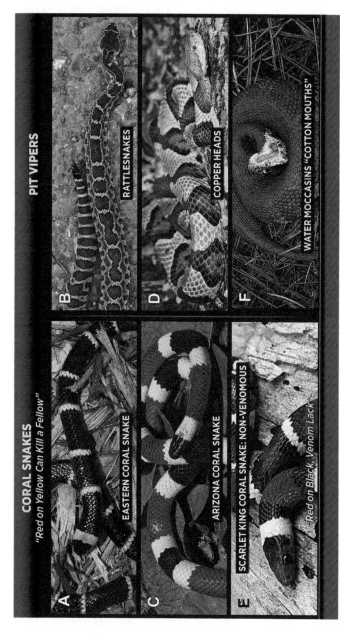

Fig. 3. Visual characteristics of venomous North American snakes. (*From* [A] Photo credit: J & T Reptiles and Exotics; [B] Photo credit: Eric Butler/National Park Service; [C] Photo credit: Jeff Servoss/USFWS; [D] Photo credit: Trisha Shears; [E] Photo credit: Glenn Bartolotti; and [F] Photo credit: CDC/ Edward J. Wozniak D.V.M., Ph.D., John Willson at the University of Georgia, at the Savannah River Ecology Laboratory [SREL].)

In contrast with the fangs among the pit vipers, coral snakes have much smaller fangs (1–3 mm vs up to 4 cm in rattlesnakes), at times leaving nearly invisible markings after envenomation. Consequently, coral snakes characteristically "chew" on the victim for a few seconds in attempt to deliver the venom, an activity that may be helpful in identification of an offending snake when not immediately known or located.[5]

Although it is certainly helpful to health care providers when exact identification of a snake responsible for envenomation is available, this is often not possible. Visual descriptions of snake characteristics are often inaccurate given the stress surrounding the encounter and brief nature of the bite. Accurate and certain identification requires either the presence of the snake at the hospital or a picture, both of which pose additional risks to the victim, bystanders, and health care providers. Additionally, envenomation by snakes thought to be dead or those who have been decapitated have been documented in the literature.[6] For individuals whose snakebite is the result of an illegal possession or handling of a snake, reluctance to share specific information, such as specific species, may be noted given fear of penalties.

ENVENOMATION

Venoms are a complex mixture of proteins, lipids, carbohydrates, and polypeptides. The exact composition, amount, and potency of venom injected is dependent on snake species, maturity, geographic location, and even the season in which the bite occurs. Significant variances in venom potency can exist within the same genus of snakes. For example, among coral snakes, the Sonoran coral snake (*Micruroides euryoxanthus*) in Arizona has a reputation for much less severe bites than the Texas coral snake (*Micruroides tener*). Generally speaking, larger snakes inject more venom. Other snake-specific variables include the number of strikes, and depth and location of the bite. Venom is most often injected subcutaneously (rather than intramuscularly or intravenously) and systemic absorption occurs via lymphatic and venous drainage of the bite site. A "dry bite," which occurs in 10% to 50%, results in a miniscule or no amount of venom being injected. Although fang markings may be noted on the skin, no local or systemic symptoms develop following extended observation.[5,7,8]

Crotalinae (Pit Viper) Envenomations

Crotalinae envenomation may include both localized and systemic symptoms. Local tissue damage is common and results in increased vascular permeability, leading to ecchymosis and progressive tissue swelling and may result in tachycardia and hypotension. Rhabdomyolysis can also be seen and, if not aggressively treated, increases the risk of acute kidney failure. Crotaline venom contains both procoagulant and anticoagulant properties, with anticoagulant effects. Thrombocytopenia is not uncommon, although serious bleeding is rare. A few species, such as the Mojave rattlesnake (*Crotalus scutulatus*) and Southern Pacific rattlesnake (*Crotalus halleri*) of California, have venom components that act on the presynaptic terminals to inhibit acetylcholine release, and may produce neurotoxic effects, such as weakness, cranial nerve dysfunction, and respiratory paralysis.[9,10]

When considering all venomous North American Crotalinae species, the venom from a rattlesnake is responsible for the greatest morbidity and mortality. Most often, the rattlesnake envenomation presents with localized soft tissue injury, but the possibility for systemic alterations and symptoms surpasses that of other species. Cottonmouth and copperhead bites are generally less severe than rattlesnake bites, and it is rare that copperhead bites lead to injuries beyond soft tissue swelling.

Elapid (Coral Snake) Envenomations

Although coral snake bites do not cause local tissue injury, cardiovascular compromise, or coagulopathies, they present a serious risk following envenomation, given the tendency for neuromuscular weakness. Although some neurotoxic effects can be seen among select Crotalinae snakes (as described previously), the more potentially serious neurologic complications (including respiratory arrest) may be seen with the coral snake and may take several hours to initially present. Particularly concerning symptoms that may indicate potential airway compromise are dysphagia, stridor, fasciculations, and muscle weakness. Although total resolution of these symptoms is possible, intubation and mechanical ventilation may be required, in some instances for prolonged time periods. Less severe abnormalities include slurred speech, paresthesias, ptosis, and diplopia.

TREATMENT

Although evidence-based guidelines are the focus of current practices, much of the prehospital treatment of snakebites remains likely to be rooted in folklore or outdated, unsupported practices. In fact, more than half of the Internet Web sites evaluated in a recent study contained inaccurate recommendations for initial care of venomous snake bites.[11] Inappropriate, and potentially harmful, interventions, such as incising the bite site, suctioning the wound, use of electrical shocks, and ice application, were all identified on Internet sites as recommended treatments of venomous snake bites.[11,12] Instead, interventions supported by research as detailed in this article should be implemented. Although developed specific to pit viper management, **Fig. 4** summarizes the overall assessment and treatment of patients following snake bite envenomation. The algorithm does not hold true, however, for coral snake bites, in which antivenom, if available, should be given for suspected and proven coral snake bites.

Prehospital Care

Interventions to slow venom spread should be implemented. Simple measures, such as keeping the patient calm and quiet, will decrease cardiac output and slow the potential spread of the venom. Jewelry on a bitten extremity should be removed in anticipation of swelling, and any tightly fitted clothing should likewise be loosened or removed. As the vast number of venomous bites in North America are of a Crotalinae etiology, with predominate soft tissue injury, use of tourniquets and pressure bandages have been shown to be even further damaging to tissues and are no longer recommended.[8,11] In fact, use of tourniquets, which occlude blood flow, may actually worsen the tissue damage by increasing distal edema and ischemia. Application of ice has also been shown to extend the local tissue injury and should be avoided.[11] Immobilizing effected extremities in a functional or extended position may prove beneficial. Hand bites should be elevated once splinted to prevent dependent edema.[5,8,13] If splints are applied, it is important to maintain vigilant assessments of the distal neurovascular status as well as the skin. Any pressure points should be padded to prevent skin breakdown.

Initial Resuscitation

On a patient's arrival to a medical facility, nursing care should immediately address airway protection, and ventilatory and hemodynamic support. Elective intubations should be considered in patients with bites to the face or neck, or those with evolving angioedema. Intravenous (IV) fluid boluses via large-bore catheters should be initiated

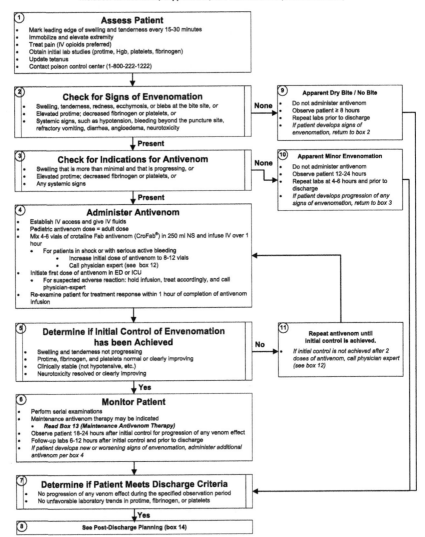

Fig. 4. Management of snakebite algorithm. (*From* Lavonas EJ, Ruha AM, Banner W, et al. Unified treatment algorithm for the management of crotaline snakebite in the United States: results of an evidence-informed consensus workshop. BMC Emerg Med 2011;11:2.)

before evidence of hypotension. Management of shock should include continued IV fluid boluses and consideration of vasopressor infusions titrated as needed. Laboratory studies, including complete blood count, metabolic profiles, liver function tests, urinalysis, and coagulation studies (prothrombin time, fibrinogen level, and platelets) should be obtained on arrival as a baseline for future monitoring.

While anaphylaxis from a snake envenomation is rare, suspicion for anaphylaxis should occur in the setting of hypotension. Prior exposure to Crotalinae venom may predispose the patient to a potential anaphylactic reaction following the

⑫
When to Call a Physician-Expert

Direct consultation with a physician-expert is recommended in certain high-risk clinical situations:

- **Life-threatening envenomation**
  Shock
  Serious active bleeding
  Facial or airway swelling
- **Hard to control envenomation**
  Envenomation that requires more than 2 doses of antivenom for initial control
- **Recurrence or delayed-onset of venom effects**
  Worsening swelling or abnormal labs (protime, fibrinogen, platelets, or hemoglobin) on follow-up visits
- **Allergic reactions to antivenom**
- **If transfusion is considered**
- **Uncommon clinical situations**
  Bites to the head and neck
  Rhabdomyolysis
  Suspected compartment syndrome
  Venom-induced hives and angioedema
- **Complicated wound issues**

If no local expert is available, a physician-expert can be reached through a certified poison center (1-800-222-1222) or the antivenom manufacturer's line (1-877-377-3784).

⑮
Treatments to <u>Avoid</u> in Pit Viper Snakebite

- Cutting and/or suctioning of the wound
- Ice
- NSAIDs
- Prophylactic antibiotics
- Prophylactic fasciotomy
- Routine use of blood products
- Shock therapy (electricity)
- Steroids (except for allergic phenomena)
- Tourniquets

⑯
Notes:

- **All treatment recommendations in this algorithm refer to crotalidae polyvalent immune Fab (ovine) (CroFab®).**
- This worksheet represents general advice from a panel of US snakebite experts convened in May, 2010. No algorithm can anticipate all clinical situations. Other valid approaches exist, and deviations from this worksheet based on individual patient needs, local resources, local treatment guidelines, and patient preferences are expected. **This document is not intended to represent a standard of care.** For more information, please see the supporting manuscript, available at: http://www.biomedcentral.com/content/pdf/1471-227X-11-2.pdf.

⑬
Maintenance Antivenom Therapy

- Maintenance therapy is additional antivenom given after initial control to prevent recurrence of limb swelling
  - Maintenance therapy is 2 vials of antivenom Q6H x 3 (given 6, 12, and 18 hours after initial control)
- Maintenance therapy may not be indicated in certain situations, such as
  - Minor envenomations
  - Facilities where close observation by a physician-expert is available.
- Follow local protocol or contact a poison center or physician-expert for advice.

⑭
Post-Discharge Planning

- Instruct patient to return for
  - Worsening swelling that is not relieved by elevation
  - Abnormal bleeding (gums, easy bruising, melena, etc.)
- Instruct patient where to seek care if symptoms of serum sickness (fever, rash, muscle/joint pains) develop
- Bleeding precautions (no contact sports, elective surgery or dental work, etc.) for 2 weeks in patients with
  - Rattlesnake envenomation
  - Abnormal protime, fibrinogen, or platelet count at any time
- Follow-up visits:
  - Antivenom not given:
    - PRN only
  - Antivenom given:
    - Copperhead victims: PRN only
    - Other snakes: Follow up with labs (protime, fibrinogen, platelets, hemoglobin) twice (2-3 days and 5-7 days), then PRN

Fig. 4. (*continued*)

development of immunoglobulin E antibodies to venom. Although sensitization occurs most commonly after venom exposure from a snake bite, antibody development has also been observed among snake handlers in whom the snake proteins are either inhaled or encountered via skin contact.[5] *Anaphylaxis resulting from a snakebite should be treated the same as classical anaphylaxis, as antivenom will not reverse this condition.* The presence of pruritus, urticaria, and/or wheezing should alert the provider to possible anaphylaxis, as these signs and symptoms are rare with uncomplicated envenomations.

History and Physical

Following the initial assessment and support of vital functions, a complete history should be obtained as the condition allows. Determining if envenomation occurred (and if so, its severity) is a priority assessment. A complete physical examination should be performed, with detailed attention to the vital signs and systems in which complications are anticipated: cardiovascular, respiratory, neurologic, and hematologic. Distal neurovascular and ongoing skin assessments should also be closely monitored in the extremity or area of the bite. Objective classification of snakebite severity is not clearly delineated and various scales have been described for this purpose. Rather than attempting to identify a particular point of severity on an evolving continuum, nursing and medical care should focus on management of the patient's symptoms, whatever they may currently be.

Generally, following an envenomation, patients experience only mild systemic symptoms (eg, nausea, nonspecific weakness) in addition to any localized symptoms. General systemic complaints may include nausea/vomiting, paresthesias, pain, diaphoresis, and tender lymphadenopathy proximal to the bite (a reliable sign of envenomation). Nonspecific symptoms, such as restlessness, anxiety, tachycardia, nausea, and abdominal pain, must not be dismissed as a stress reaction without thorough investigation, as they may signify systemic envenomation. Depending on the location of bite and manner of distribution (lymphatic vs intravascular), systemic symptoms may be delayed in onset. However, in the most extreme presentations, patients may initially present with hypovolemic shock or airway compromise especially in the presence of significant comorbidities or facial/neck bites.

Swelling and pain with an extremity bite may develop within minutes of a significant crotaline envenomation and can progress rapidly and extensively. Atypical presentations with delay in initial swelling up to 10 hours has been reported, most often with bites on the lower extremities.[5] For this reason, any edema or erythema borders should be outlined with pen or marker and circumferential measurements obtained above and below the bite site. Close monitoring for advancement should occur every 15 to 30 minutes.[8,13]

Wound Care

Snake bite wounds should be considered contaminated puncture wounds and treated accordingly. Goals of wound care following envenomation are aimed at limiting tissue damage. Basic wound care including irrigation of the wound with saline solution or tap water should be performed. Because povidone-iodine and hydrogen peroxide solutions are now known to be toxic to tissues and may delay wound healing, they should not be used.[14,15]

Hemorrhagic blisters (or "blebs") commonly occur within hours following rattlesnake bites, and may progress over several days. Similar to burns, large blebs may require debridement for evaluation of underlying tissues and to relieve pain associated with pressure from the lesions. Although healthy tissue is typically found underneath, widespread distribution may represent more extensive underlying necrosis and may ultimately warrant surgical debridement (although this is rare).[5,8] Necrosis of the digits after a finger or toe strike may lead to need for significant debridement or amputation. This is a rare complication, occurring 1 to 2 weeks following envenomation, rather than in the initial period if it indeed does occur.

Observation

For patients with suspected bites from a North American crotaline snake in whom no initial physical alterations are seen, observation for at least 8 to 12 hours remains prudent. Shorter observation periods of 4 to 6 hours may be acceptable in the setting of known copperhead bites.[5] When suspected envenomation results from an exotic or foreign species, increasing the period of observation up to 24 hours is recommended. Patients with a potential coral snake bite are recommended to undergo a minimum of 24-hour observation given the high likelihood for rapid and severe clinical deterioration. If no symptoms are seen at the end of this time frame, it can be assumed that a patient has sustained a dry bite with no envenomation.

When evidence of envenomation is recognized, longer observation and more aggressive treatments are typically required. If only mild, localized symptoms (pain and swelling) with no evidence of laboratory abnormalities, patients may be admitted for a 24-hour observation on telemetry. Intensive care admissions are warranted for those patients who experience progressive local symptoms (eg, swelling that progresses beyond the immediate bite area or who develop tissue necrosis) or any systemic symptoms. In these patients, analgesic medications, IV fluids, hemodynamic monitoring, and routine laboratory assessments comprise the basis of care in addition to the wound care discussed previously. Ventilatory and hemodynamic support in the form of oxygen and vasopressors may be required. Progression of symptoms may require the use of full ventilatory support, although this is very rare.

Medications

Overall, the medications used in treatment of patients status-post envenomations are similar to those frequently used in critical care areas and emergency departments. As with all wounds, tetanus immunization status must be assessed and updated as needed. If the vaccination history is unknown or the patient received fewer than 3 initial doses, a tetanus vaccine and tetanus immune globulin should be given. If a complete 3-injection series was initially completed, tetanus vaccination alone should be given if the last dose was longer than 5 years prior.[14,15] For adults who have not received a dose of tetanus-diphtheria-pertussis vaccine (Tdap), this formulation may be used rather than the tetanus-diphtheria vaccine (Td).[16]

Analgesics and sedatives play particularly predominate roles among patients requiring critical care following envenomation. Opioid medications, given intravenously, are commonly used for pain management.[13] For patients requiring mechanical ventilation, sedation will likely be required for tolerance of the ventilation mode, as well as for control of symptoms of restless and psychomotor agitation.

As infections at the bite site are uncommon, antibiotic therapy is reserved for cases with evidence of cellulitis or other localized infections.[8,13]

Antivenoms

In very general terms, antivenoms are produced by inoculating animals (typically sheep or horses) with venom from particular species and then collecting and processing the serum from the immunized animal. Single or multiple species can be used for the immunization, producing either a monospecific (from 1 species) or polyspecific (more than 1 species) antivenom. With particular regard to snake antivenoms, the most ideal antivenom is polyspecific, including the venom from multiple species of snakes indigenous to the geographic area where the antivenom is most likely to be used.

Of all snake envenomations that occur in the United States, approximately 70% receive antivenom.[17] The decision to administer antivenom must be considered on a case-by-case basis. Before administration, contraindications described by the manufacturer should be explored and considered. *It is highly recommended that the local poison control center and/or a medical toxicologist be consulted before using antivenom.*

Use in Crotalinae envenomation

Treatment with antivenom is reserved for cases of moderate to severe envenomation presenting with systemic symptoms and laboratory abnormalities. Indications for administration of antivenom following a Crotalinae envenomation include hemodynamic compromise, significant coagulopathy or thrombocytopenia, neuromuscular toxicity, or progressive swelling. Antivenom is not indicated for anaphylaxis, and should not be given as prophylaxis.

Effective administration of antivenom is time sensitive. Timely administration of antivenom, once it is determined that the patient needs it, has been shown to reduce the duration and severity of coagulopathies and thrombocytopenia and to prevent local swelling progression. Local tissue necrosis, however, is not prevented by antivenom. Additionally, antivenom will not reverse any tissue damage that has already occurred.

There is only one antivenom currently available for administration following North American pit viper envenomations: Crotalidae polyvalent immune Fab (CroFab). The sheep serum–derived antivenom is composed of a mixture of venom from 4 commonly encountered North American pit vipers, and is administered intravenously. As the antivenom is ovine-derived, previous reactions to equine-derived antivenoms is not a contraindication. Medications for resuscitation in the event of hypersensitivity or anaphylactic reactions should nevertheless be immediately available. If such a reaction does occur, the antivenom infusion must be stopped and the patient given IV steroids, histamine antagonists, epinephrine, and fluid boluses, as necessary. In patients at high risk for profound morbidity and mortality following envenomation, the antivenom infusion is only then restarted at much lower doses and given concurrently with epinephrine infusions.[5,18]

Dosing of the antivenom is dependent on patient symptomatology, and most often requires repeated dosing. Detailed dosing and reconstitution instructions accompany the antivenom and should be followed. An initial dose of 4 to 6 vials is mixed with normal saline solution and infused intravenously at a slow rate. If no signs of anaphylaxis develop, the infusion rate is increased to achieve completion within 1 hour. Following completion of the initial dose, the patient should be reassessed for worsening swelling, thrombocytopenia, or coagulopathy. If these are identified, then an additional 4-vial to 6-vial dose should be infused. Repeated infusions and reassessments are continued until resolution of the symptoms occurs. Once the patient's symptoms have stabilized or improved, assessments of advancing erythema or swelling may be slowed to repeat measurements every 1 to 2 hours. Additionally, 1 maintenance dose (consisting of 2 vials of antivenom in 250 mL of 0.9% normal saline given over an hour) should be administered every 6 hours for a total of 3 maintenance doses. Repeated maintenance doses are required, as the antivenom half-life is shorter than that of the venom. Failure to continue treatment with the maintenance doses may result in return of swelling, coagulopathies, or thrombocytopenia. Despite appropriate maintenance therapy, it is not uncommon for some patients to develop recurrence of abnormal laboratory studies 3 to 4 days following the antivenom treatments, thus follow-up at this time is important.

With envenomation of the pregnant woman, fetal demise approaches 50%, whereas maternal deaths are rare. Data from the AAPCC support safe administration of CroFab antivenom to pregnant women, with no short-term documented adverse reactions, maternal deaths, or fetal demise.[19] In contrast, others report fetal death rates nearing 60% in mothers given antivenom.[20] Conflicting case studies and systematic reviews provide no clear consensus regarding management of snakebites in the pregnant woman. In such cases, expert guidance from a medical toxicologist/poison center should be sought expediently to evaluate each situation independently.

Use in Elapidae envenomation
It is suggested that any patient with confirmed coral snake bite or skin penetration receive antivenom, even in the absence of symptoms. Unfortunately, the last lot of Elapidae antivenom expired on October 31, 2012. It is reported that production will begin again in 2013. Treatment following coral snake envenomation is then left to supportive measures only.

COMPLICATIONS

Complications, such as compartment syndrome, rhabdomyolysis, and coagulopathies, must be anticipated.

Compartment Syndrome

Evaluation for developing compartment syndrome is difficult, as the expected effects of the venom, such as paresthesias, significant swelling, muscle weakness, and pain with passive stretching, may mimic signs of compartment syndrome. Crotaline envenomation classically causes local tissue injury with significant destruction of underlying tissues; however, given the size of the fangs of the Crotalinae snake, it is uncommon for the fascia to be penetrated with the bite, and thus the notable swelling occurs outside of the subfascial compartments. Compartment pressures need to be obtained if compartment syndrome is suspected, but findings must be interpreted carefully. Elevated intracompartmental pressures have been documented following Crotalinae envenomation, even in settings without clear evidence of compartment syndrome or hypoperfusion.[21] Very rarely, fasciotomies may be required, but they are by no means the initial standard of care. When performed, fasciotomies should be performed only in the setting of documented elevations in compartment pressures and clinical evidence of hypoperfusion. Nonsurgical approaches, such as extremity elevation as possible and administration of antivenom, may circumvent the need for fasciotomy. In fact, recent studies support the use of antivenom over fasciotomy for reduction of intracompartmental pressures to improve tissue perfusion.[2,21,22]

Rhabdomyolysis

Rhabdomyolysis can occur with or without an accompanying compartment syndrome, and has been described following envenomations from a variety of snake species. Resulting from muscle necrosis, rhabdomyolysis is characterized by release of intracellular muscle contents (eg, electrolytes, myoglobin, creatine kinase) into the circulation. If untreated, rhabdomyolysis can lead to acute kidney injury, so ongoing surveillance for its development is crucial. Although elevations in total serum creatine kinase (directly resulting from muscle necrosis), reddish-brown discoloration of urine (evidence of myoglobinuria), and myalgias are clinical indicators of rhabdomyolysis, diagnosis is made based on the creatine kinase levels.[23,24] Routine assessments of pain, urine output, and appearance, as well as total serum creatine kinase levels, are crucial for surveillance.

If it develops, rhabdomyolysis must be treated aggressively to avoid acute kidney injury. Electrolyte abnormalities, including hyperkalemia and hypocalcemia should be anticipated in the setting of rhabdomyolysis, and should therefore be assessed frequently and treated appropriately should they develop. The cornerstone of treatment is early and aggressive isotonic IV fluids in hopes to flush the large protein molecules through the kidneys and prevent acute injury. Urine output should be maintained at 3 mL/kg per hour. Alkalinization of urine and use of mannitol remain controversial but may be used in some settings.[24]

Coagulopathies

Of the Crotalinae snakes, rattlesnake envenomations pose the greatest risk on the hematologic system. Following a moderate to severe envenomation, fibrinogen levels may drop to near zero with a platelet count that can plummet to the 10,000–50,000/mm[3] range. In addition, a high prothrombin time (greater than 100 seconds) may be seen following Crotalinae envenomation. Despite these alterations, most patients do not experience any bleeding even in the case of severe laboratory abnormalities; however, on discharge, patients should be cautioned about the risks of bleeding from an accident (ie, falling of a roof). The same advice should be given to patients with snakebite as to those on anticoagulation therapy until their follow-up shows a normal hematologic profile. Disseminated intravascular coagulation with multisystem organ failure is rarely seen, but has been reported following intravascular envenomation.[5,25]

Administration of blood products should be reserved for those patients who exhibit clinically significant bleeding.[13] Because the venom causing the bleeding abnormalities is still present when the infusions are given, transfused blood products will likely be similarly affected by the venom and rendered unhelpful. Patients with active bleeding who require blood products should receive concurrent doses of antivenom. In most cases, correction of coagulopathies, thrombocytopenia, and any mild bleeding can be achieved with the appropriate use of antivenom.

OUTCOMES

Overall, deaths and severe tissue necrosis requiring amputation are exceptionally rare among North American envenomations. Access to specialized medical care is almost always available within the first few hours, likely improving morbidity and mortality among this population. The poorer outcomes that are documented are almost always attributable to delay in receiving medical care or envenomation from a more dangerous, nonindigenous species.

In patients who develop rhabdomyolysis with subsequent acute kidney injury requiring dialysis, long-term renal sequela may include continued proteinuria, hypertension, and chronic kidney disease. Some of these patients will eventually progress to develop end-stage renal disease requiring long-term dialysis.[26] However, most patients experiencing acute kidney injury secondary to rhabdomyolysis ultimately recover renal function and long-term survival in these patients nears 80%.[24]

SCORPION ENVENOMATIONS

Among arachnids worldwide, scorpion envenomation is the leading cause of morbidity and mortality, especially in children.[27] Within the United States there is only one species of scorpions responsible for medically significant envenomations: *Centruroides sculpturatus,* more commonly referred to as the "bark scorpion."[28] The bark scorpion is a nocturnal small, yellow-brown arachnid with 8 legs, typically only 4.0 to 7.5 cm in length. The sharp distal tip of the segmented tail (referred to as the "telson") is responsible for envenomation.

The 2011 Annual Report of the AAPCC indicated just over 19,000 calls regarding potential scorpion envenomations. Of these, roughly 900 resulted in significant morbidity, although there were no deaths reported. Although envenomations have been reported in Southern California, Utah, Nevada, and New Mexico, they are most concentrated within Arizona and northern Mexico.[29] Given that the higher incidence of scorpion stings occur per capita in Mexico, the more diverse scorpion population, and the close proximity to the United States, some of these patients may present for care within US facilities as well.

Venom

Similar to snake venom, scorpion venom is a complex mixture of many components and toxins that bind to the voltage-gated sodium, potassium, chloride, and calcium channels. It is thought that resulting alterations in the action potential are primarily responsible for the neurotoxic effects of the bark scorpion venom.[30]

Clinical Manifestations

Severe pain occurs with all scorpion stings regardless of species. The pain is usually localized and almost always occurs within 1 hour of the sting, often accompanied by paresthesias of the affected limb, and may persist for up to 30 hours.[31] Although pain always occurs, edema does not, which is a unique characteristic of scorpion envenomation that may prove helpful in distinguishing from snake bites.

Systemic effects of envenomation from the bark scorpion are multifactorial, dependent on the venom potency, volume injected, and patient weight. The effects are predominately neurotoxic, manifesting as ataxia, restlessness/agitation, tremors, and tongue fasciculations. Oculomotor abnormalities may also occur, including opsoclonus: rapid, involuntary, and multivectorial eye movements. Parasympathetic stimulation may also occur, resulting in hypersalivation, lacrimation, and vomiting.[28,32,33]

Physical examination focuses on the sting area and identification of any neurologic symptoms, as described previously. Unique to envenomation by the bark scorpion, pain is intensified by tapping over the area of the sting. This finding may help distinguish a scorpion envenomation from other envenomations.

Treatment

Given the short-lived duration of symptoms, which are rarely life-threatening, supportive care and pain management constitute the basis of treatment. The onset of symptoms following scorpion envenomation is immediate, with peak severity usually appearing within 4 to 6 hours. Resolution of symptoms may take up to 30 hours.[32] Hospitalization in adults is rarely required, but may be necessary in young children or others with signs of systemic toxicity, or in patients whose pain cannot be controlled initially.

As pain associated with scorpion stings is usually severe, parenteral analgesics are frequently required. Sedation with benzodiazepines may be required in situations of profound abnormal muscular excitation and agitation.[28] As in any situation in which opioids and benzodiazepines are used concurrently, or in large doses, the nurse must pay close attention to the patient's respiratory status. In pediatric patients, sedative medications may also be used at lower doses as adjunctive therapy for pain management.

The use of atropine to reverse excessive oral secretions is controversial in the management of parasympathetic effects of scorpion stings. Although some studies have shown it to be a benefit in hypersalivation, it may also exacerbate sympathetic effects, and for this reason should be reserved for treatment of severe bradycardia.[34,35] Tetanus prophylaxis should be updated based on the patient's immunization status.

Antivenom

The use of antivenom in *Centruroides* envenomations is controversial. Although morbidity may be severe, the risk of death even without treatment remains much lower than the risk for anaphylaxis from antivenom administration. Recently approved by the Food and Drug Administration in 2011, *Centruroides* (scorpion) Immune F(ab') 2 (Anascorp; Accredo Health Group, Inc., Memphis, TN) is the only scorpion-specific antivenom available in the United States. The scorpion antivenom contains animal serum–derived immunoglobulins, in partial fragments, which bind directly to and interrupt the toxic functions and have been shown to be effective in reversing neurotoxicity from *Centruroides* scorpion evenomation.[28,33,36]

Nonexperimental observations and controlled studies alike have repeatedly noted faster resolution of neurotoxicity symptoms with the use of scorpion-specific antivenom.[28,33] In critically ill pediatric patients with significant neurotoxic effects, use of the scorpion-specific antivenom has been associated with symptom resolution within 4 hours, a reduced need for sedative infusions, and decreased levels of plasma venom.[28]

Recommendations for antivenom therapy following a *C. Sculpturatus* sting are not clearly defined. Most commonly, use is reserved for cases in which systemic toxicity presents in the form of cranial nerve or skeletal muscle abnormalities. The decision for antivenom use in such envenomations is best reached in conjunction with a medical toxicologist.

IMPLICATIONS FOR NURSING PRACTICE

Given the complexity of care of patients following envenomation, outcomes may be enhanced with incorporation of a multidisciplinary team. Medical toxicologists should be contacted early in the assessment and treatment through the local poison center. Surgical consults (in particular, hand surgeons as indicated) should be requested for evaluation of necrosis and need for debridement. Specialists in nephrology may be involved in the setting of rhabdomyolysis, and pulmonology should ventilator management be required. Early involvement from physical and/or occupational therapy can help to mobilize fluid, prevent development of joint contractures, and reduce deconditioning in the critically ill individual. Case management may be beneficial in arranging outpatient follow-up 3 to 5 days after antivenom therapy is complete to provide laboratory reassessment for possible recurrent abnormalities. Critical care nurses are uniquely positioned to play a vital role in coordinating the clinical care of patients following envenomation.

As the world's borders become blurred because of increase of travel and immigration, health care providers must maintain awareness of initial treatment of envenomations. For the instances in which a bite or sting occurred in a geographically remote area from that of patient presentation, or in the case of bites from exotic, non-native species, collaboration with other providers will be essential. Experts from the geographic region in which the envenomation occurred will likely prove helpful, if the ability for contact and conversation are possible. Regional Poison Centers (1-800-222-1222) remain available to collaborate in treatment planning and procuring available antivenoms.

ACKNOWLEDGMENTS

The authors acknowledge Keith Wood and Dina Bahan, both of Vanderbilt University School of Nursing, for their graphic artwork expertise in development of illustrations for this article.

REFERENCES

1. Bronstein AC, Spyker DA, Cantilena LR, et al. 2011 Annual Report of the American Association of Poison Control Centers' National Poison Data System (NPDS): 29th Annual Report. Clin Toxicol (Phila) 2012;50:911–1164.
2. Walker JP, Morrison RL. Current management of copperhead snakebite. J Am Coll Surg 2011;212:470–5.
3. Cruz NS, Alvarez RG. Rattlesnake bite complications in 19 children. Pediatr Emerg Care 1994;10:30–3.
4. Seifert SA, Boyer LV, Benson BE, et al. AAPCC database characterization of native U.S. venomous snake exposures, 2001-2005. Clin Toxicol (Phila) 2009; 47:327–35.
5. Riley BD, Pizon AF, Ruha AM. Snakes and other reptiles. In: Nelson L, Lewin N, Howland MA, et al, editors. Goldfrank's toxicologic emergencies. 9th edition. New York: McGraw-Hill; 2010. p. 1601–15.
6. Suchard JR, LoVecchio F. Envenomations by rattlesnakes thought to be dead. N Engl J Med 1999;340:1930.
7. Gold BS, Dart RC, Barish RA. Bites of venomous snakes. J Emerg Med 2002;347: 347–56.
8. Madsen W, Elfar J. Snake bites. J Hand Surg Am 2010;35:1700–2.
9. Bush SP, Siedenburg E. Neurotoxicity associated with suspected southern pacific rattlesnake (*Crotalus viridis helelri*) envenomation [Erratum appears in Wilderness Environ Med 2000;11:226]. Wilderness Environ Med 1999;10:247–9.
10. Jansen PW, Perkin RM, Stralen DV. Mojave rattlesnake envenomation: prolonged neurotoxicity and rhabdomyolysis. Ann Emerg Med 1992;21:322–5.
11. Barker S, Charlton NP, Holstege CP. Accuracy of Internet recommendations for prehospital care of venomous snake bites. Wilderness Environ Med 2010;21: 298–302.
12. Seifert S, White J, Currie BJ. Pressure bandaging for North American snake bite? No! Clin Toxicol (Phila) 2011;49:883–5.
13. Lavonas EJ, Ruha AM, Banner W, et al. Unified treatment algorithm for the management of crotaline snakebite in the United States: results of an evidence-informed consensus workshop. BMC Emerg Med 2011;11:2. http: //dx.doi.org/10.1186/1471-227X-11-2.
14. Nick BA, Ayello EA, Woo K, et al. Acute wound management: revisiting the approach to assessment, irrigation, and closure considerations. Int J Emerg Med 2010;3:399–407.
15. Agency for Healthcare Research and Quality, National Guideline Clearinghouse. Management of human bite wounds. 2007. Available at: http://www.guideline.gov/content.aspx?id=10860&search=human+bite+wounds. Accessed December 21, 2012.
16. Wolfe RM. Update on adult immunizations. J Am Board Fam Med 2012;25: 496–510.
17. Weinstein S, Dart RC, Staples A, et al. Envenomations: an overview of clinical toxinology for the primary care physician. Am Fam Physician 2009;80:793–802.
18. Spiller HA, Bosse GM, Ryan ML. Use of antivenom for snakebites reported to United States poison centers. Am J Emerg Med 2010;28:780–5.
19. LaMonica GE, Seifert SA, Rayburn WF. Rattlesnake bites in pregnant women. J Reprod Med 2010;55:520–2.
20. Langley RL. Snakebite during pregnancy: a literature review. Wilderness Environ Med 2010;21:54–60.

21. Cumpston KL. Is there a role for fasciotomy in Crotalinae envenomations in North America? Clin Toxicol (Phila) 2011;49:351–65.
22. Gold BS, Barish RA, Dart RC, et al. Resolution of compartment syndrome after rattlesnake envenomation utilizing non-invasive measures. J Emerg Med 2003; 24:285–8.
23. Miller ML. Clinical manifestations and diagnosis of rhabdomyolysis. Available at: www.uptodate.com. Accessed December 26, 2012.
24. Bosch X, Poch E, Grau JM. Rhabdomyolysis and acute kidney injury. N Engl J Med 2009;361:62–72.
25. Curry SC, Kunkel DB. Toxicology rounds. Death from a rattlesnake bite. Am J Emerg Med 1985;3:227–35.
26. Waikhom R, Sircar D, Patil K, et al. Long-term renal outcome of snake bite and acute kidney injury: a single-center experience. Ren Fail 2012;34:271–4.
27. Isbister GK, Volschenk ES, Seymor JE. Scorpion stings in Australia: five definitive stings and a review. Intern Med J 2004;34:427–30.
28. Boyer LV, Theodorou AA, Berg RA, et al. Antivenom for critically ill children with neurotoxicity from scorpion stings. N Engl J Med 2009;360:2090–8.
29. Cheng D, Dattaro JA, Yakobi R. Scorpion envenomation. Emedicine. Available at: http://emedicine.medscape.com/article/168230. Accessed December 21, 2012.
30. Zhijian C, Yingliang W, Jiqun S, et al. Evidence for the existence of a common ancestor of scorpion toxins affecting ion channels. J Biochem Mol Toxicol 2003;17:235–8.
31. Rimsza ME, Zimmerman DR, Bergeson PS. Scorpion envenomation. Pediatrics 1980;66:298–302.
32. Hahn I, Clark RF. Arthropods. In: Nelson L, Lewin N, Howland MA, et al, editors. Goldfrank's toxicologic emergencies. 9th edition. New York: McGraw-Hill; 2010. p. 1561–87.
33. Tuuri RE, Reynolds S. Scorpion envenomation and antivenom therapy. Pediatr Emerg Care 2011;27:667–75.
34. Dehesa-Davila M, Alagon AC, Possani LD. Clinical toxicology of scorpion stings. In: Meier J, White J, editors. Handbook of clinical toxicology of animal venoms and poisons. Boca Raton (FL): CRC press; 1995. p. 221–37.
35. Thomas JD, Thomas KE, Kazzi ZN. Venomous arthropods. In: Shannon MW, Borron SW, Burns MJ, editors. Haddad & Winchester's clinical management of poisoning and drug overdose. 4th edition. Philadelphia: Saunders; 2007. p. 1601–15.
36. Anascorp [package insert]. Memphis (TN): Accredo Health Group, Inc; 2011.

West Nile Virus

An Infectious Viral Agent to the Central Nervous System

Francisca Farrar, EdD, MSN, RN

KEYWORDS

- Infectious epidemic arboviral virus • Nonneuroinvasive disease
- Neuroinvasive disease • Meningitis • Encephalitis • Acute flaccid paralysis

KEY POINTS

- The West Nile virus is a reportable arboviral illness.
- The primary route of human infection is by an incidental bite of a mosquito carrying the infection.
- Infected immune cells can transport the virus to the central nervous system.
- Potential complications from neuroinvasive disease include meningitis, encephalitis, and acute asymmetric flaccid paralysis.
- Critical care nursing management is supportive therapy and symptom management.
- Prevention is the key to elimination of the West Nile virus, because there is no vaccine.

INTRODUCTION

Summer is a time for vacations and exploring the outdoors. Outdoor summer activities expose people to unwanted accidents, such as tick and mosquito bites. The black-legged deer tick can cause Lyme disease, whereas the American dog tick and the Rocky Mountain wood tick can cause Rocky Mountain spotted fever. A mosquito bite can infect a person, causing them to develop the West Nile virus (WNV). A person with WNV can be asymptomatic, develop mild flulike symptoms, or develop a neuro-invasive infection that can cause meningitis, encephalitis, or acute flaccid paralysis, requiring the patient to be admitted to the critical care unit for treatment.[1] A WNV vaccine with effectiveness in horses has been licensed, but a WNV vaccine for humans is still not available.[1] The WNV has emerged as an important global virus, causing epidemics and viral encephalitis.[1] This article focuses on the WNV as a summer accident.

School of Nursing, Austin Peay State University, McCord, Room 218, PO Box 4658, Clarksville, TN 37044, USA
E-mail address: farrarf@apsu.edu

Crit Care Nurs Clin N Am 25 (2013) 191–203
http://dx.doi.org/10.1016/j.ccell.2013.02.005
0899-5885/13/$ – see front matter © 2013 Elsevier Inc. All rights reserved.

ccnursing.theclinics.com

The WNV is a single-stranded RNA virus of the family Flaviviridae, genus *Flavivirus*, and a member of the Japanese encephalitis virus antigenic complex.[2,3] The WNV is one of the most widely distributed arboviruses, with incidences reported in Africa, the Middle East, parts of Europe, the former Soviet Union, South Asia, Australia, United States, Canada, Latin America, and the Caribbean.[3] The WNV was first discovered in Uganda in 1937.[4] The first case was discovered in the United States in New York City in 1999.[4] The WNV caused 62 cases of encephalitis and 7 deaths in New York during this discovery time.[3] Since 1999, the WNV has been detected in 48 continental states, the District of Columbia, and Puerto Rico.[3] In North America, the WNV has established a seasonal epidemic pattern in association with proliferation of mosquito populations, with peak incidence occurring between July and October.[1] Transmission is year round in temperature climates such as the southern United States.[1]

SURVEILLANCE PROGRAM AND STATISTICS

WNV is an arboviral illness declared to be reportable because it is dangerous to the public. All physicians, hospitals, laboratories, health care providers, and any person knowing or suspecting WNV are responsible for reporting it to the health department.[5] Local and state health departments in the United States are required to submit surveillance and statistical reports to the Centers for Disease Control and Prevention (CDC). The electronic surveillance reports are submitted to a national database called Arbo-Net.[6] The CDC generates a map of incidence by states and a WNV case report by states in the United States. CDC statistical data were used for the development of **Tables 1** and **2**.[6] The statistics in **Table 1** point out a surge of WNV cases over the last 4 years. As of October 23, 2012, ArboNet reported that neuroinvasive disease cases outnumbered noninvasive disease cases. Deaths from complications from WNV also statistically grew.

Data analysis of **Table 2** reveals that California, Mississippi, and Texas were listed in the top 4 states with the highest reported WNV cases in 3 of the 4 year reports. As of October 23, 2012, Texas data document an epidemic of WNV in the state, with 1628 reported WNV cases with 743 neuroinvasive cases, 885 nonneuroinvasive cases, and 74 deaths. As of October 23, 2012 data also show that 48 states reported WNV cases, with a total of 4725 cases including 2413 neuroinvasive cases, 2312 nonneuroinvasive cases, and 219 deaths.

TRANSMISSION

The primary route of human infection of WNV is through the bite of a mosquito carrying the infection. The WNV is not transmitted through person-to-person contact. Transfused blood and transplanted organs are less common routes of WNV.[3] Infection

Table 1
WNV human infections reported to ArboNet, United States, 2009–2012

Year	Neuroinvasive Disease Cases	Nonneuroinvasive Disease Cases	Total Cases	Deaths
2009	373	322	720	32
2010	629	329	1021	57
2011	486	226	712	43
2012	2413	2312	4725	219

Note: 2012 statistics reported as of October 23, 2012.

Table 2
Top 4 states with WNV human infections reported to ArboNet, United States, 2009–2012

Year	Top Four States	Neuroinvasive Disease Cases	Nonneuroinvasive Disease Cases	Total Cases	Deaths
2009	Texas	93	22	115	9
	California	63	45	112	4
	Colorado	36	67	103	3
	Mississippi	31	22	53	5
2010	Arizona	107	60	167	31
	New York	89	39	128	16
	California	72	39	111	6
	Texas	77	12	89	6
2011	California	110	48	158	9
	Arizona	49	20	69	4
	Mississippi	31	21	52	5
	New York	28	16	44	2
2012	Texas	743	885	1628	74
	Mississippi	97	136	233	5
	California	198	128	326	15
	Louisiana	118	121	239	11

Note: 2012 statistics reported as of October 23, 2012.

via breastfeeding and from pregnant mother to baby has occurred in a few cases.[1,2] The mosquito transmission cycle is as follows:

- Birds act as reservoirs. The virus circulates in nature through an enzootic cycle in which the infection remains steady between wild birds and domestic birds.[1] Wild birds serve as amplifying hosts by developing prolonged high levels of viremia. Surveillance of dead birds, especially crows, ravens, and jays, is associated with incidences of WNV.[3]
- Mosquitoes are the primary vector. Adult mosquitoes acquire the WNV by feeding on the blood of infected birds and inoculate the virus in their saliva.[1,3] Thereby, the mosquito becomes a carrier of the virus. Mosquitoes breed in fresh water habitats such as temporary pools of waters, and proliferate during humid, warm seasons.[1] Surveillance has identified 64 mosquito species infected with the WNV.[2,3] The most common genus that transmits the WNV is *Culex*.[2,3]
- Humans get infected incidentally when exposed to the infected mosquito. The mosquito bites the individual during a feeding process and the mosquito injects WNV-laden saliva into the human, with dissemination occurring.[1,3] The virus replicates in skin Langerhans dendritic cells, and infected cells migrate to regional lymph nodes. The lymph nodes can spread viremia seeds to various organs and tissues such as liver and kidney. Infected immune cells can transport the virus to the central nervous system, putting the patient at risk for neuroinvasive disease such as severe meningitis and encephalitis.[3]

CLINICAL MANIFESTATIONS

Approximately 1 in 5 people infected with the WNV present with symptoms such as fever, headache, malaise, back pain, myalgias, anorexia, vomiting, and rash.[7] A patient with WNV typically develops symptoms between 3 and 14 days after being bitten by an infected mosquito.[1,2] Potential complications of WNV are encephalitis, meningitis, or an acute asymmetric flaccid paralysis. These severe neuroinvasive diseases occur in approximately 1 in 150 cases.[8] Encephalitis is more commonly reported than meningitis.[8] People older than 50 years and those with medical conditions such as cancer, diabetes, hypertension, kidney disease, and organ transplants and immunosuppressed patients are at risk for development of neuroinvasive clinical manifestations.[3,8] Clinical disease ranges from mild febrile illness to severe encephalitis.[9] The WNV is categorized into 2 primary groups: neuroinvasive disease and non-neuroinvasive disease.

Nonneuroinvasive Disease

In nonneuroinvasive disease, the WNV replicates in the body but not in the central nervous system.[5] In nonneuroinvasive disease, the patient may present asymptomatic or develop the following major clinical manifestations:

- West Nile fever is a self-limited illness persisting from 3 to 6 days. The patient presents with fever, headache, malaise, back pain, myalgias, and anorexia. Other flulike symptoms include pharyngitis, nausea, vomiting, diarrhea, and abdominal pain. Eye pain can also occur. Some patients may present with a low-grade fever or no fever with the West Nile fever clinical manifestations.[10]
- Approximately 50% of patients develop a maculopapular rash.[10] West Nile rash is typically maculopapular and generally lasts less than 1 week. The maculopapular rash can be associated with dysesthesia and pruritis. The rash involves the chest, back, and arms.[10]
- Fatigue is the most persistent symptom, lasting an average of 36 days. This persistent symptom leads to missed work and a patient's inability to perform activities of daily living.[10]

Neuroinvasive Disease

In neuroinvasive disease, the patient begins with early flulike symptoms with a brief febrile syndrome. The symptoms progress in severity as the WNV replicates within the central nervous system, causing inflammation in the brain and spinal cord.[5] The patient can present with fever, lethargy, altered mental status, incoordination, abnormal reflexes, paresis/paralysis, convulsions, and stiff neck,[5] Complications such as respiratory failure and death can occur. The following is an overview of clinical manifestations that the patient with neuroinvasive disease may develop:

- Encephalitis is a neuroinvasive disease complication, which ranges from mild to severe. In mild encephalitis, the patient presents with a self-limited confusion state. In severe encephalitis, coma and death can occur.[10] Clinical diagnosis of encephalitis is associated with older age, alcohol abuse, and diabetes.[10]
- Viral meningitis can occur. Signs and symptoms usually begin suddenly with a temperature up to 40°C (104°F), drowsiness, confusion, stupor, slight stiff neck or spine stiffness when bending forward, and headache.[11]
- Extrapyramidal symptoms are commonly associated with WNV. Other clinical manifestations include course tremor and myoclonus, especially in the upper extremities. Parkinsonian signs and symptoms such as rigidity, postural instability, and bradykinesia are also associated with WNV.[10]
- Acute flaccid paralysis is a neuroinvasive disease complication, which can lead to respiratory failure. The asymmetric paralysis results from an anterior horn cell process, suggesting poliomyelitis.[10] Cranial nerve palsy is a potential clinical manifestation resulting in facial weakness, vertigo, dysarthria, and dysphagia.

Cranial nerve palsy combined with acute flaccid paralysis puts the patient at risk for respiratory failure.[10]
- Seizures, cerebellar ataxia, and optic neuritis are less common neurologic complications.[10]
- Ocular signs and symptoms include chorioretinitis, retinal hemorrhages, vitritis, iridocyclitis, occlusive vasculitis, and uveitis producing persistent visual deficit. Optic neuritis and occlusive vasculitis can induce permanent visual deficit.[10]
- Less common complications of WNV include rhabdomyolysis, fatal hemorrhagic fever with multiorgan failure with palpable purpura, hepatitis, pancreatitis, central diabetes insipidus, myocarditis, myositis, and orchitis.[10]

DIAGNOSTIC TESTS

A patient with a sudden onset of unexplained fever, encephalitis, meningitis, or flaccid paralysis during mosquito season needs diagnostic evaluation. Laboratory testing for antibody production in response to the WNV viremia can confirm the WNV diagnosis. A WNV IgM antibody-capture enzyme-linked immunoassay of serum or cerebrospinal fluid (CSF) collection is the gold standard diagnostic test.[1] A lumbar puncture to evaluate the cerebral spinal fluid, imaging, and electroencephalography (EEG) can confirm neuroinvasive complications from the WNV diagnosis.[10] The following is an overview of common diagnostic tests to confirm the WNV diagnosis:

- WNV triggers increased antibody production in response to West Nile viremia. Testing for the detection of IgM antibody to WNV is recommended within the first 8 days of illness.[10] Plasma samples are tested for WNV RNA by transcription-mediated amplification and for WNV-specific IgM and IgG, which rapidly develop after viremia.[10] Serologic testing is recommended. The nucleic acid amplification test used for blood donor screening can be used for severely immunocompromised patients, who may lack IgM antibody, or complement serologic testing, if urgent diagnosis is required.[10] The IgM antibody to WNV may persist for 6 months are longer.
- Patients infected with WNV can have false-positive antibody testing as a result of recent immunizations, such as yellow fever or Japanese encephalitis.[10]
- A lumbar puncture and assessment of the cerebral spinal fluid for the detection of IgM antibody for pleocytosis is recommended for a patient with WNV neuroinvasive clinical manifestations. In pleocytosis, there is a predominance of lymphocytes and increased protein levels.[10] Glucose level is normal.[1]
- Imaging is recommended for a patient with altered mental status and suspected neuroinvasive disease. Computed tomography of the brain and spinal cord shows poor sensitivity in cases with neuroinvasive disease.[1] Magnetic resonance imaging (MRI) is abnormal in cases of meningitis and encephalitis showing signs of meningeal inflammation and bilateral lesions.[1] MRI usually shows abnormal patterns of increased signal intensity in the brain regions such as the basal ganglia, thalmi, and caudate nuclei. Hyperintensity is also seen in the brainstem and spinal cord.[10]
- EEG is recommended with patients with neuroinvasive signs and symptoms such as meningitis, acute flaccid paralysis, and encephalitis.[10] EEG typically shows generalized continuous slowing with patients with generalized meningitis or encephalitis that is more prominent in the temporal or frontal regions.[10] In patients with acute flaccid paralysis, EEG shows widespread fibrillation potentials and compound motor action potentials, depending on the degree of paralysis, varying between normal and marked decreased activity.[10]

CLINICAL SYNDROMES OF MENINGITIS VERSUS ENCEPHALITIS

A central nervous system infection caused by the WNV can result in clinical syndromes of meningitis and encephalitis. The presence or absence of normal brain function is the important differentiation feature between them.[12] A patient with viral meningitis has normal cerebral function, whereas a patient with encephalitis has abnormalities in brain function. The clinical presentation of viral meningitis includes fever, headache, nausea/vomiting, photophobia, and stiff neck The patient with encephalitis has altered mental status, motor or sensory deficits, altered behavior and personality changes, and speech or movement disorders.[12] The patient with encephalitis may have additional neurologic signs and symptoms, such as hemiparesis, flaccid paralysis, and paresthesias.[12] Seizures are common with encephalitis.[12] The patient may have clinical features of both and is diagnosed based on which clinical features predominate in the illness.[12]

West Nile Meningitis

Meningitis is an inflammation of the protective membrane surrounding the brain and spinal cord, which can include the pia mater, arachnoid, the CSF-filled subarachnoid space, and the dura mater.[13] West Nile viremia causes aseptic meningitis, which does not require isolation of the patient.

Pathophysiology

West Nile viremia violates the protective covering of the brain and spinal cord. The host immune response results in an inflammatory response in the involved meninges. The inflammatory responses cause an increased viscosity of the CSF, which can interfere with CSF absorption, which can result in increased intracranial pressure, cerebral edema, and hydrocephalus.[13]

Clinical manifestations

Headache and high fever are the initial symptoms. Nuchal rigidity (stiff neck) is an early sign in 30% to 70% of patients.[13] The patient can present with normal mental status or with an altered level of consciousness with disorientation and memory impairment, which can progress depending on severity of the illness to lethargy, unresponsiveness, and coma. Seizures can occur.[13] Initial signs of increased intracranial pressure (ICP) include decreased level of consciousness and focal motor deficits. Vomiting is also a sign of increasing ICP.[13]

Meningitis Case Report

JC is an active 74-year-old female survivor of breast cancer who lives alone. She presented to the emergency room with complaints of a headache, neck pain, and back pain, which was rated 7/10. JC also complained of nausea, vomiting, and malaise. She reported that these flulike symptoms had been progressive for 3 days. She was alert and oriented × 3. Her temperature was 38.3°C (101°F). JC's chest radiograph was normal along with a normal urinalysis. Her white blood count was slightly increased. She was diagnosed with a viral infection and discharged home with orders for rest, fluids for hydration, and acetaminophen plus propoxyphene (Darvocet) for pain. JC was instructed to follow up with her primary care physician as needed. The next day her daughter went to check on JC. The daughter found JC confused with a temperature of 40°C (104°F). JC was crying that her neck hurt and no one would help her. The daughter called the primary doctor to report clinical findings and the deterioration of JC. The doctor asked the daughter to bring JC to her office immediately. JC required a wheelchair when she was taken to the doctor's office because of extreme weakness and lethargy. JC required sunglasses while en route to the doctor because of photophobia. On examination, the doctor was suspicious that JC had viral meningitis. JC was admitted directly to the hospital, with an order for a lumbar puncture. The CSF confirmed viral meningitis. The history revealed that JC was working in a garden by a creek in her backyard before her illness. The daughter reported that JC complained that the mosquitoes were "bad" because of a recent rainstorm and she had been bitten by mosquitoes several times while working in her garden. The doctor ordered a polymerase chain reaction assay for antibody titers to test for WNV antibody production, and the CSF was also tested for WNV. Both tests were positive for the WNV. The physician diagnosed JC with West Nile meningitis.

This meningitis case report shows classic West Nile meningitis progression. JC began with mild flulike symptoms that progressed to neuroinvasive signs and symptoms of meningitis, which included high fever, severe headache, vomiting, photophobia, and stiff neck. JC was elderly and a cancer survivor, who had had recent chemotherapy and radiation therapy, which placed her at higher risk for developing meningitis. JC also had an exposure to a mosquito bite. JC's treatment was symptom focused. Medical management was ordered for treatment of fever, pain, and increased ICP. The room was kept dark for her photophobia. JC was admitted to a neurologic critical care unit for neurologic observation, assessment, and treatment to prevent further complications.

West Nile Encephalitis

The WNV is the most common type of arboviral encephalitis and elderly people are at increased risk.[13]

Pathophysiology

When the mosquito bites a human, viral replication occurs and the person's immune system is triggered to control viral replication. If the immune system fails, viremia occurs. The virus continues to replicate until it reaches the central nervous system via the cerebral capillaries, causing encephalitis. The virus spreads from neuron to neuron, affecting primarily the cortical gray matter, the brainstem, and the thalamus. Exudate from the meningeal irritates the meninges and increases the ICP.[13]

Clinical manifestations

Viral encephalitis begins with early flulike symptoms, with a brief febrile prodrome. Signs and symptoms specific to West Nile encephalitis include maculopapular rash on the neck, trunk, arms, and legs. Flaccid paralysis is also a clinical manifestation. Encephalitis can cause Parkinsonian-like movements. Seizures are a poor prognosis.[13] MRI shows inflammation in the periventricular area. IgM antibodies to WNV are found in serum and CSF. Blood cultures are not useful, because the viremia is brief.[13]

Encephalitis Case Report

BF, a 69-year-old diabetic male with 3 days of flulike symptoms of nausea, vomiting, malaise, anorexia, and a rash, was found in bed by his spouse confused, lethargic, and with a fever of 39.4°C (103°F). The spouse called the emergency response system. BF was taken to the local emergency room. In the emergency room, the patient became combative, requiring haloperidol (Haldol) for sedation. BF's chest radiograph was normal, along with normal blood glucose levels and urinalysis. The white blood count was increased. Blood cultures were pending. MRI results were abnormal, with inflammation in the periventricular area. The patient was life-flighted to a certified neurointensive care unit for further evaluation and treatment. In route to the neurointensive care unit, the patient vomited and was intubated for airway protection. On arrival at the neurointensive care unit, a seizure was witnessed and he was given intravenous lorazepam (Ativan). The patient was placed on a mechanical ventilator, because he was already intubated. During his neurologic examination, it was discovered that he had acute flaccid paralysis in the left lower leg. A bedside lumbar puncture was performed with CSF analysis, showing pleocytosis with a predominance of lymphocytes, normal glucose, and increased protein levels. EEG showed marked decreased activity of motor action potentials and areas of fibrillation potentials. A history revealed that the patient had been on a camping trip with his spouse for 1 week before becoming ill. The spouse reported that mosquitoes were a problem at the campsite and the patient had been bitten by mosquitoes several times. A polymerase chain reaction assay for antibody titers was ordered for WNV antibody production, and the CSF was tested for WNV. Both tests were positive for the WNV. The physician diagnosed BF with West Nile encephalitis with acute flaccid paralysis as a complication.

This encephalitis case report shows classic West Nile encephalitis progression. The patient began with febrile flulike symptoms, which progressed to neuroinvasive signs and symptoms. The neuroinvasive disease clinical manifestations were altered mental status, acute flaccid paralysis, seizure, and the abnormal MRI. BF was an older, diabetic patient, which placed him at higher risk for developing encephalitis. He also had multiple exposures to mosquito bites. His treatment was symptom focused. Medical management was ordered for controlling the increased ICP, supporting respiratory function, and controlling the seizures.[13] Antibiotic therapy was not justified because this was a viral infection. The neurointensive care unit placement was appropriate for specialty neurologic observation, assessment, and treatment required in an attempt to prevent complications that can lead to death or lifelong neurologic deficits and seizures.[13]

CRITICAL CARE NURSING MANAGEMENT OF WNV NEUROINVASIVE DISEASE

Treatment of WNV is supportive and based on signs and symptoms and clinical presentation. **Table 3** gives an overview of supportive therapy considerations and critical care nursing management of a patient with the complication of neuroinvasive disease from WNV:

Risk Factors

Identification of people at risk for becoming infected with WNV is important. These high-risk individuals are in need of education and interventions for prevention. Outdoor exposure in areas where there is activity of WNV increases their risk of mosquito bites and WNV infection. The risk for neuroinvasive disease increases in people aged 50 years and older, and patients with cancer or kidney disease, diabetes, or who are immunocompromised.[1] The following are examples of high-risk groups:

- Persons older than 50 years: surveillance data identify that persons older than 50 years are at higher risk for severe disease and death.[19] Data also correlate a relationship between risk and patients with cancer or kidney disease, diabetes, and who are immunocompromised.[1] Activities such as jogging, golf, and gardening can expose them to mosquito bites.[19] Education can prevent WNV in this group.
- Persons with outdoor exposure: people employed in outdoor work or engaged in recreational activities outdoor are at a greater risk of being bitten by WNV-infected mosquitoes. Insect repellent and protective clothes can help prevent mosquito bites in this group.[19]

- Homeless persons: this high-risk group has extensive outdoor exposure and limited financial resources. Social service can provide resources to this high-risk group if contacted.[19]
- Persons who live in residences lacking window screens: the lack of protective screens is a risk factor for exposure to mosquito bites. Community organizations such as churches and service groups can help with repairing and obtaining screens.[19]

Prevention

Prevention is the key to elimination of WNV in humans via mosquito bites. The following is an overview of preventive measures:

- Seasonal surveillance depending on geographic region. Surveillance of avian morbidity/mortality, mosquitoes, and human cases can prevent the transmission of WNV. The following outlines these 3 important areas of surveillance:
  - Avian morbidity/mortality: the American crow is the most sensitive species for avian morbidity/mortality surveillance in northern regions in the United States. Early detecting and ongoing monitoring of dead birds infected with WNV helps health officials predict and prevent human infection.[19] Dead birds provide the earliest detection of WNV activity in an area. People should be educated to report dead birds and not to touch or handle a dead bird, because of the risk of exposure to WNV.
  - Mosquitoes: mosquito surveillance is a primary tool for quantifying the intensity of WNV transmission in an area. Adult mosquitoes and larval mosquitoes are collected and screened for WNV. Trapped mosquitoes provide information about virus infection rates, vector species, and quantifiable information on potential risk to humans, and allow evaluation of control methods.[19]
  - Surveillancehuman cases: national reporting of WNV to ArboNet allows the CDC to develop statistical data to identify the local, state, and national impact of WNV. Data document the need for public health intervention programs, need for allocated resources, and identification of high-risk populations. Monitoring of encephalitis cases is a priority.[19]
- Personal protection measures: avoid accidental mosquito bites by the use of insect repellants. Use insect repellents containing an Environmental Protection Agency–registered insect repellent.[1,4,20] N,N-Diethyl-meta-toluamide (commonly known as DEET), picaridin, IR3535, or lemon-eucalyptus repellent are insect repellants recommended by the state health department.[5,20] Wearing long sleeves and trousers tucked into boots or shoes when mosquitoes are most active at dusk and dawn can also prevent a mosquito bite.
- Source reduction: simple activities can reduce mosquito breeding habitats. Examples of source reduction activities include emptying standing water in buckets, old tires, birdbaths, flowerpots, pet dishes, unused swimming pools, and cleaning gutters.
- Mosquito control programs: insecticides can be directed against the immature or adult stage of the mosquito life cycle. Chemicals used comply with state and federal requirements. Public health pesticide applicators are required to be licensed or certified by the appropriate state agency.[19] Truck-mounted or aerial insecticide spraying in communities with heightened human infection risk identified by mosquito surveillance programs kills mosquito larvae and adult mosquitoes.[18,19] Insecticide spraying has minimal pesticide exposure and associated insecticide-related illness.[4]

Table 3
Supportive therapy considerations for WNV

Problem	Nursing Management
Altered LOC	Assess for signs and symptoms of neuroinvasive disease Assess neurologic status for changes Use neurologic tool such as Glasgow Coma Scale, which assesses patient's response to stimuli. Scores range from 15 (normal) to 3 (deep coma) Assess for deterioration and improvement Assess verbal response to orientation to person, place, and time Assess papillary response for evidence of neurologic disease and decline Assess for complications of acute flaccid paralysis, cranial nerve palsy, extrapyramidal symptoms, and Parkinsonian signs and symptoms
Altered respiratory function	Assess respiratory status Provide supplemental oxygen to keep oxygen saturation 92% and higher Continuous monitoring of oxygen saturation Prevent aspiration because patient is high risk as a result of decreased LOC Keep HOB 30° and put patient in sitting position for feeding if able to eat Assess need for protective airway management with intubation and mechanical ventilation for vomiting, decreased LOC, and respiratory failure Assess arterial blood gases as needed to determine respiratory status and need for respiratory support Assess for respiratory failure in patient with complication of acute flaccid paralysis or cranial nerve palsy
Altered cardiovascular status	Assess circulatory status with cardiac monitoring to assess for arrhythmias Assess blood pressure for adequate perfusion to body and brain Arterial line if needed to monitor arterial pressures Central line for fluid management and central venous pressure readings with evaluation Use a pulmonary artery catheter if needed for circulatory management
Dehydration and electrolyte problems	Interpret complete blood counts and electrolytes Correct electrolyte imbalances Hydrate per orders Avoid overhydration especially if patient has cerebral edema
Cerebral edema	Assess for signs and symptoms of cerebral edema Administer osmotic diuretics such as mannitol, which is gold standard Maintain parameters for mannitol by obtaining scheduled serum sodium and osmolarity levels Enforce fluid restrictions Administer intravenous corticosteroid if ordered to decrease inflammation
Fever	Assess temperature for abnormality Follow protocol for temperature more than 38.9°C (102°F) with chest radiograph, blood cultures, and urinalysis per physician's order to rule out secondary bacterial infection Administer antipyretics such as acetaminophen as ordered. Suppository can be given per rectum for decreased LOC or liquid per tube if needed Place patient on hypothermia blanket with continuous temperature monitoring Run fan on low in room to lower body temperature Keep cover to minimum Administer cool bath

(continued on next page)

Table 3 (continued)	
Problem	**Nursing Management**
Increased ICP	Assess for deterioration in level of consciousness and vomiting as signs of increased ICP
	Continuous ICP monitoring via intraventricular catheter with hourly readings
	Keep HOB at 30° at all time
	If order for CSF to drain to decrease ICP, measure every hour along with pressure readings and assess drainage
Seizures	Assess for seizure including time, type, and behavior involved
	Administer anticonvulsant medications such as phenytoin (Dilantin) and levetiracetam (Keppra) if ordered
	Administer intravenous lorazepam (Ativan) if ordered
	Implement seizure precaution protocol
Viral infection	Educate patient and family about WNV
	Administer supportive drug therapy for WNV ordered by physician such as acyclovir, interferon α, and immunoglobulin intravenously
	Implement standard infection control measures
	Enforce strict handwashing for staff, family, and visitors
	Report WNV case to local state health department per hospital and state policy
Neuropsychiatric complications	Assess for neuropsychiatric complications such as agitation, emotional outbursts, and combative behavior
	Administer chemical constraints such as Haldol as ordered
	Implement restraint protocol for physical constraint
	Maintain quiet environment
	Limit visitation
	Referral for psychiatric consultation if needed
Photophobia in meningitis	Assess for signs and symptoms of photophobia
	Darken room and keep bright lights out of room
	Implement safety measures with light restriction
Pain	Assess for signs and symptoms of pain
	Implement pain management program including comfort measures
	Administer analgesics for headache and pain
	Administer opiates as ordered
Nutritional needs	Assess nutritional status
	Assess ability to swallow and risk for aspiration for per mouth feeding
	Request speech evaluation if needed
	Provide feedings per Dobbhoff tube or Flexiflo feeding tube if ordered
	Nutritional consult for caloric needs, order for tube feeding, or need for total parenteral nutrition
	Keep HOB 30°
Mobility impairment	Implement fall precautions
	Implement measures to prevent pressure areas and to prevent decubitus ulcers
	Facilitate order for physical therapy and occupational therapy
	Follow activity orders per physician such as chair for 2 h 3 times a day or bed chair
Rehabilitation need	Case management referral for discharge needs such as skill facility rehabilitation, home health care, or need for placement outside of home
	Provide discharge information to patient and family regarding support groups and resources available in community

Abbreviations: HOB, head of bed; LOC, level of consciousness.
Data from Refs[13–18] and personal experience as a neurointensive care critical care nurse.

- Blood donor screening programs: screening of donated blood reduces the risk of transfusion transmission. WNV infection should be ruled out in a patient with unexplained signs and symptoms of WNV after a recent blood transfusion.[18]
- Vaccine development: equine WNV vaccines have been licensed in the United States, but there is no vaccine for humans. Research for a vaccine is being conducted.[18]

SUMMARY

The WNV is a reportable arboviral illness, which has emerged as an important global virus, which may cause epidemics. The primary route of human infection is through an incidental bite of a mosquito carrying the infection. As of October 23, 2012 in the United States, the CDC surveillance data showed 48 states reporting WNV cases, with a total of 4725 cases, including 2413 neuroinvasive cases, 2312 noninvasive cases, and 219 deaths. A person with WNV can be asymptomatic, develop flulike symptoms, or develop a neuroinvasive infection, which can cause meningitis, encephalitis, and acute flaccid paralysis. A patient with WNV may have clinical features of both meningitis and encephalitis. The presence or absence of normal brain function is the important differentiation feature between them. Case reports show the differences between the 2 clinical syndromes. Critical care nursing management is based on symptom management and supportive therapy for neuroinvasive disease complications. Critical care nursing management for complications includes altered level of consciousness, mechanical ventilator respiratory support, high fever, cerebral edema, increased ICP, seizures, and neuropsychiatric issues. Prevention is the key to elimination, such as surveillance programs, personal protective measures, source reduction, mosquito programs, and vaccine development.

REFERENCES

1. Centers for Disease Control and Prevention. West Nile Virus (WNV) fact sheet. Available at: http://www.cdc.gov/westnile. Accessed May 16, 2012.
2. Centers for Disease Control and Prevention. West Nile Virus: epidemiologic information for clinicians. Available at: http://www.cdc.gov/westnile. Accessed May 16, 2012.
3. Peterson LR, Hirsch MS, McGovern BH. Epidemiology and pathogenesis of West Nile virus infection. Available at: http://www.uptodate.com. Accessed May 16, 2012.
4. Peterson LR, Hirsch MS, McGovern BH. Patient information: West Nile virus infection (beyond the basics). Available at: http://www.uptodate.com. Accessed May 16, 2012.
5. Tennessee Department of Health. Arboviral illness. Available at: http://health. state.tn.us/ReportableDiseases/ReportableDiseases.aspx/HealthcareDescription. Accessed September 7, 2012.
6. Centers for Disease Control and Prevention. Statistics, surveillance, and control. Available at: http://www.cdc.westnile. Accessed September 7, 2012.
7. Centers for Disease Control and Prevention. West Nile virus disease cases up this year. Press release. Available at: http://www.cdc.westnile. Accessed October 29, 2012.
8. Centers for Disease Control and Prevention. Fact sheet: West Nile Virus (WNV) infection: information for clinicians. Available at: http://www.cdc.westnile. Accessed October 29, 2012.

9. Centers for Disease Control and Prevention. Arboviral diseases, neuroinvasive and non-neuroinvasive. Available at: http://www.cdc.gov/osels/ph_surveillance/nndss/print/arboviral_current.htm. Accessed September 7, 2012.

10. Peterson LR, Hirsch MS, McGovern BH. Clinical manifestations and diagnosis of West Nile virus infection. Available at: http://www.uptodate.com. Accessed May 16, 2012.

11. Eckman M, Share D. Neurologic disorders. In: Pathophysiology made incredibly easy. Philadelphia: Lippincott Williams & Wilkins; 2013. p. 143–8.

12. Johnson RP, Gluckman SJ. Viral encephalitis in adults. Available at: http://www.uptodate.com. Accessed October 29, 2012.

13. Bautista C. Nursing management: patients with neurologic disorders. In: Pellico LH, editor. Focus on adult health medical-surgical nursing. Philadelphia: Lippincott Williams & Wilkins; 2013. p. 1218–22.

14. Baird MS, Bethel S. Neurologic disorders. In: Manual of critical care nursing: nursing interventions and collaborative management. St Louis (MO): Mosby; 2011. p. 644–51.

15. Hinkle JL, et al. Neurologic function. In: Smeltzer SC, Bare BG, Hinkle JL, editors. Brunner & Suddarth's textbook for medical-surgical nursing. Philadelphia: Lippincott Williams & Wilkins; 2010. p. 1954–55.

16. Zomorodi M. Acute intracranial problems. In: Lewis SL, Dirksen SR, Heitkemper MM, et al, editors. Medical surgical nursing: assessment and management of clinical problems. St Louis (MO): Elsevier Mosby; 2011. p. 1455–7.

17. Bautista C. Nursing management: patients with neurologic disorders. In: Pellio LH, editor. Focus on adult health medical-surgical nursing. Philadelphia: Lippincott Williams & Wilkins; 2013. p. 1221–2.

18. Peterson LR, Hirsh MS, McGovern BH. Treatment and prevention of West Nile virus infection. Available at: http://www.uptodate.com. Accessed May 16, 2012.

19. Centers for Disease Control and Prevention. Epidemic/epizootic West Nile Virus in the United States: guidelines for surveillance prevention, and control. Available at: http://www.cdc.gov. Accessed May 16, 2012.

20. Breisch NL, Golden DB, Feldweg AM. Prevention of arthropod and insect bites: repellents and other measures. Available at: http://www.uptodate.com. Accessed October 29, 2012.

Spider Envenomation in North America

Richard S. Vetter, MS[a,b,*]

KEYWORDS

- Envenomation • Spider • Latrodectism • Loxoscelism • Necrotic arachnidism
- Methicillin-resistant *Staphylococcus aureus*

KEY POINTS

- Spider bites are perceived to be a greater detriment to human health than in actuality, with only the widow and recluse groups causing medically important bites in North America.
- Widow spider bites cause systemic reactions involving the muscle and nervous systems, with few dermatologic signs; a large percentage of these bites results in moderate to severe reactions.
- Recluse spider bites cause dermatologic damage and, in rare cases, systemic reactions, but most recluse bites are minor and self-healing.
- Many medical conditions result in dermonecrotic lesions that can be or have been misdiagnosed as recluse spider bites.
- Bacterial infections, especially methicillin-resistant *Staphylococcus aureus*, have often been mistaken for recluse spider bites, but with growing awareness in recent years skin lesions are being more accurately diagnosed than in previous decades.

INTRODUCTION

Spiders occupy an interesting position in human society and in medicine. The overall health risk that they pose is minor compared with other routine events such as driving an automobile, vocational and recreational hazards, or living an unhealthy lifestyle. Yet the psychological aspects of their existence, including arachnophobia or arachno-adverse reactions, coupled with the dynamic nature of envenomation, give the condition of "spider bite" an elevated importance and newsworthiness in North America. Although most spider bites are of little concern, on rare occasions severe envenomations can lead to serious disease or even death. Accurate diagnosis and proper supportive care are crucial in reducing the morbidity associated with spider envenomations.

Disclosure Statement: The author has nothing to disclose.
[a] Department of Entomology, University of California, Riverside, Riverside, CA 92521, USA;
[b] Division of Biological Sciences, San Bernardino County Museum, 2024 Orange Tree Lane, Redlands, CA 92374, USA
* Department of Entomology, University of California, Riverside, Riverside, CA 92521.
E-mail address: rick.vetter@ucr.edu

At present, there are only 2 medically important groups of spiders in North America: the widow spiders and the recluse spiders. Other species have historically been implicated in human disease, but have been shown to be erroneously blamed (yellow sac spider) or their venom toxicity is currently in doubt (hobo spiders). In addition, in the last decade or so there have been 2 significant improvements in envenomation toxicology and patient care. One is the spotlight focused on the many causes of dermonecrosis that are misdiagnosed as brown recluse spider bites, and the other is the recognition of community-acquired methicillin-resistant *Staphylococcus aureus* (MRSA) as a common cause of skin and soft-tissue injury that mimics a severe bite from a brown recluse spider. Bringing to light these issues has significantly reduced the erroneous attribution of necrotic skin lesions to spider bites.

DEFINITIONS

When discussing spiders and bites, it is important to define the terms under consideration. One of the most common errors is the synonymous use of the words "bites" and "stings." A bite is inflicted with a hardened structure (fang, teeth) from the oral end of the body, whereas a sting is inflicted with the posterior end of the body. Spiders and snakes bite. Honey bees, wasps, and scorpions sting. Honey bees can also bite but it is their sting that is painful.

Other common terms that are misused include the words "venomous," "poisonous," and "toxic." Venomous merely describes an anatomic situation whereby an organism has a venom gland, ductwork, and a hardened apparatus for injecting a subdermal load of venom. Venomous does not connote physiologic effect, although by its nature it does have a target organism. Some snakes and most spiders are venomous. Poisonous describes the anatomic situation of possessing a poison gland that secretes a substance but not through ducting. Poison generally just exudes from a gland or covers a body part, and is effective when ingested or delivered topically. Poison-arrow frogs and nightshade are poisonous. To connote detrimental physiologic effect, one must use the word toxic, which means there is a consequence of the deployment of the venom or poison to the receiver of the toxin. When using the word toxic one must also include the target organism, for example, "black widow spiders have venom that is toxic to humans." This phrasing is critical when considering the example of the cobra, which is venomous by its anatomic configuration, and is toxic to humans because of the deleterious physiologic nature of its venom. However, to the mongoose, which is immune to cobra venom, the cobra is not viewed as toxic but is instead considered sustenance, as mongooses eat cobras. Hence, it is incorrect to state that a spider is venomous or poisonous to humans.

WIDOW SPIDERS
Species and Distribution

Five species of widow spiders (genus *Latrodectus*) exist in North America[1]; however, only 3 are widespread and occur in situations that place them in contact with humans such that envenomations are likely. The southern black widow (*Latrodectus mactans*) is found predominantly in the southeastern quadrant of the United States. The western black widow (*Latrodectus hesperus*) is found predominantly from the Pacific Coast to east of the Rocky Mountains, and from British Columbia south to Mexico. This distribution includes high-elevation locales with winter snow such as Denver, and low-elevation deserts with scorching heat. The brown widow (*Latrodectus geometricus*) is a nonnative species from Africa, which established itself initially in Florida and is now found across the southeastern United States from Texas to North Carolina, as well as in southern California.

Appearance

The well-known appearance of the black widow spider is that of a shiny black body and legs with a red hourglass on the belly of a globular abdomen (**Fig. 1**). However, the immatures start out life with white stripes and look very different from adult females (**Fig. 2**A).[2] Immatures gain black coloration as they mature, and the white stripes dissipate. Males are smaller in body than females, although the larger males can have leg spans that rival females. Males retain the striped coloration of the juvenile and, hence, are not often correctly identified by nonarachnologists.

Epidemiology

Widow spiders are rarely found in domestic living spaces, preferring garages, outbuildings, and outdoor locations with their webs close to the ground.[2,3] In the first half of the twentieth century, widow spider bites were common in outhouses, with many bites occurring on the genitalia and buttocks. Bite victims were predominantly men.[4] With the advent of indoor plumbing, bites shifted to the extremities when people would don gloves or boots, especially ones that had been in storage for a lengthy time. About half of the envenomations are on the lower extremities with about another quarter on the upper extremities.[5] Bites by male and immature black widow spiders may evoke symptoms, but typically are minor because of their smaller size, lower venom quantity, and weaker oral musculature such that piercing human skin is more difficult.

Symptomology and Pathophysiology

Envenomation by a widow spider is known as latrodectism. The symptoms associated with latrodectism are well known with little controversy, so almost everything involving widow bites is straightforward. The bite is either not felt or resembles a pinprick. Widow venom works on the neuromuscular junction, causing release of neurotransmitters from the presynaptic vesicles (in the absence of calcium), causing muscles to contract.[6] In addition, the venom prevents the reabsorption of the neurotransmitters back into the presynaptic vesicles, leading to prolonged stimulation of the muscle and repeated or sustained painful contractions. Onset of symptoms occurs about 1 hour after envenomation, with the bite victim most often seeking medical help within 6 hours post bite.[5] Of the 3 grades of widow envenomations presented by Clark and colleagues,[5] most patients exhibited the intermediate (37%) or high (54%) grade of signs and symptoms of latrodectism. Pain initially develops locally at the bite site, and may spread regionally in the bitten area. It may also radiate to or emanate from

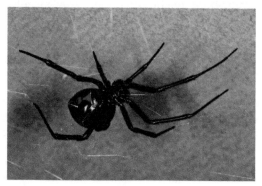

Fig. 1. Black widow spider. (Photos © R. Vetter.)

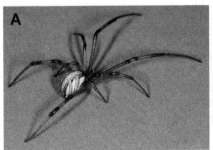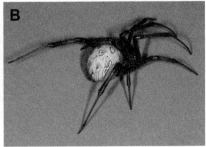

Fig. 2. Immature black widow spiders (*A*) and brown widow spiders (*B*) are frequently mistaken for one another. (Photos © R. Vetter.)

the back, chest, or abdomen. Abdominal muscles may become rigid, mimicking an acute surgical abdomen. Diaphoresis occurs and may be limited to the bite site, or may occur in unusual distribution patterns, such as below both knees, or asymmetrically in the region of the bite while the rest of the body is dry. Sweating may be profound, and in Australian widow bite victims, sweat accumulating in puddles on the floor below a bitten leg was noted.[7] Hypertension may occur. The patient is restless and moves incessantly to ameliorate pain, to the point where taking a patient's history may be difficult.[7] Muscle fasciculations and oliguria may also be present. Less commonly one may see tachycardia, nausea, vomiting, and headache.[5] There is little dermatologic indication of a bite other than erythema or a target lesion consisting of a puncture site surrounded concentrically by blanching and then erythema.[5] This lesion may be subtle and transient or could be unremarkable. The bite victim may exhibit facies latrodectismica, which consists of painful grimacing, flushing, diaphoresis, trismus, and blepharitis.[8] Although widow venom affects muscle contraction, no prenatal losses occurred in 97 pregnant bite victims.[9] Worldwide, deaths were recorded in the early twentieth century[10] but since the advent of effective medication and supportive care, deaths nowadays are rare.

Misdiagnoses

Because the bite symptoms of widow envenomation are almost pathognomonic, true widow spider bites are rarely misdiagnosed. However, cases presenting with tender, rigid abdominal muscles have been mistaken for acute abdomen (ie, appendicitis).

Treatment

In the early 1900s, remedy for widow spider bites included whiskey, cocaine, and nitroglycerine, among others.[11] Later, muscle relaxants such as calcium gluconate were used; however, these were shown to be ineffective.[5] At present, opioid and nonopioid analgesics as well as benzodiazepines are recommended for pain relief.[6] Laboratory panels are not diagnostically helpful, but certain parameters such as creatine kinase or serum creatinine may need to be measured to catch complications of serious envenomations.

Widow antivenom can completely ameliorate the effects of latrodectism within 30 minutes,[5] and appears to be effective even if given after a lengthy delay.[12] Experimentally, widow antivenom has efficacy on many *Latrodectus* species worldwide such that widow antivenom should have universal applicability.[13] Because widow antivenom is derived from horse serum, many American physicians are hesitant to use it. This concern may stem from a single case report of death via antivenom anaphylaxis in a young woman who had asthma in addition to multiple medication sensitivities, and received an undiluted dose rapidly administered.[8] Australian health practitioners use widow antivenom intramuscularly, frequently with good efficacy and rapid amelioration of severe symptoms, whereas American physicians use intravenous antivenom. However, controversy exists regarding efficacy of intramuscular versus intravenous administration and whether widow antivenom is effective at all.[6] Proper dilution and slow administration of antivenom in conjunction with close monitoring for allergic reaction should help obviate concerns about antivenom usage. As an added precaution, medications to treat anaphylaxis should be kept ready at the bedside during antivenom administration.

BROWN WIDOW SPIDERS

Brown widow spiders have been the focus of much concern over the last decade in the southern United States. The population was confined to Florida for years, but in the early twenty-first century spread from Texas to South Carolina and into southern California. Brown widows are almost strictly outdoor spiders, rarely found in homes and garages, especially if the door is usually shut.[3] However, around urban property the brown widow can be very prolific, with every patio chair and table supporting multiple specimens. Envenomation risk is greatest when spiders make their homes in recessed locations where people stick their fingers and exert pressure, such as under the curled lips of potted plants and in the grab hole of plastic trash bins.[3] Brown widows are striped throughout life and exhibit great variation, from a cream to almost black abdomen. Brown widows can readily be mistaken for immature black widows, owing to similar striping patterns (see **Fig. 2**); differentiating them from black widows requires an experienced arachnologist. Identity can much more readily be established by their egg sacs, which have silk spikes covering the surface, making the sac look like a giant pollen ball or a World War II harbor mine. By contrast, black widow egg sacs have a smooth surface.

This spider's bite is much less toxic than that of native black widows. In one series of 15 verified bites from Africa where the spider originates, the 2 most common symptoms were pain on inception and burning pain at bite site.[14] Brown widow envenomation did not have the expression of typical latrodectism. Although documented bites with more dynamic symptoms have been recorded,[15–17] general supportive care should be sufficient for most brown widow bites.

FALSE BLACK WIDOWS

The false black widow, Steatoda grossa, is of European origin and is found in many areas of the United States, especially the Pacific coast and in the southeastern states. It is a combfoot spider similar to widow spiders, and is chocolate brown in color with no red coloration on its ventral abdomen. It is slightly smaller than an adult widow and is readily mistaken for a black widow by nonarachnologists.

It is not uncommonly involved in envenomations because, unlike black and brown widows, it is often found inside homes. Its bite is like that of a mild black widow envenomation.[18] In one case in Australia, red back widow antivenom was administered for a false black widow bite, with reported symptomatic relief.[19]

RECLUSE SPIDERS
Species and Distribution

Thirteen species of recluse spider (genus Loxosceles) occur in North America, 2 of which are nonnatives.[20] The brown recluse (Loxosceles reclusa) is found predominantly in the Midwestern United States; 5 other species have wide distribution in the south-western United States (**Fig. 3**). The Mediterranean recluse (*Loxosceles rufescens*) is a worldwide tramp species, which is found very rarely around the United States (and only inside buildings). The Chilean recluse (*Loxosceles laeta*) is established in some locations in urban Los Angeles County but mostly in the basements of commercial buildings, not in homes. Despite its potent venom, it is not considered a health issue by county department of health entomologists because of its lack of interaction with humans.

Despite the insistence of many nonarachnologists, recluse spiders are not found throughout North America, they are not expanding their range, and they are rare or nonexistent over much of the continent.[20] Although a recent Geographic Information System study modeled their potential spread north with global warming,[21] recluse spiders do not disperse readily.[20] If global warming has an effect, an equally tenable scenario to northerly expansion is that the spiders might become extinct in the southern portion of their range and may not be able to expand northward, hence reducing both their current distribution and envenomation threat.

Appearance

Brown recluse spiders are typically unremarkably tan colored with a brown violin shape on the front portion of the body (cephalothorax) (**Fig. 4**). However, because nonarachnologists are very creative in interpreting violins on all surfaces of spider bodies, rampant misidentifications occur.[22,23] For example, male crevice weaver spiders (genus *Kukulcania*) (**Fig. 5**) are routinely submitted as brown recluses from the southern third of the United States where, even with a dead spider in hand and availability of comparison images on the Internet, nonarachnologists (including physicians) envision this spider having a violin marking.[22,23] In addition, many south-western American recluse spiders have no pigment in the violin area and, hence, resemble generic tan spiders.

The most reliable way to identify a recluse spider is to examine the eye pattern. Most spiders have 8 eyes arranged in 2 or 3 rows. Recluse spiders have 6 eyes arranged in pairs in a backward facing U-shape. A pair of eyes occurs in front and a pair on either side, with spaces between the pairs (**Fig. 6**). A few other spiders have this eye pattern, but the leg and abdominal coloration is spotted or striped in these species as opposed to the recluse's monochromatic coloration.

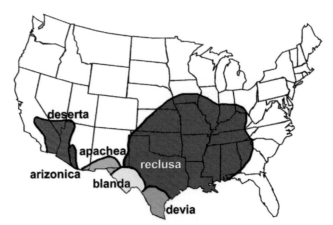

Fig. 3. Distribution map of recluse spiders in America. (Photos © R. Vetter.)

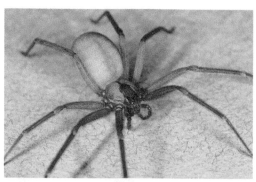

Fig. 4. Brown recluse spider. (Photos © R. Vetter.)

Epidemiology

Recluse envenomations typically occur when the spider is trapped against human flesh and inflicts a bite as a last-ditch defensive response. Recluse bites are generally undetected or felt as a minor pinprick. Most bites occur when people are putting on clothes or shoes that have laid on the floor overnight, or when they roll over onto a spider while sleeping. Bites are most frequently recorded on the legs, followed in frequency by bites to the arms, torso, and, rarely, the face (**Table 1**). South American research showed that female recluse spider venom caused larger lesions in rabbits than did the venom of males, leading to the conclusion that female recluse venom may be more potent.[24,25] Recluse spiders follow a seasonal periodicity in North America, with spiders being found almost exclusively in the warm months, even inside heated homes.[26] Diagnoses of recluse bite reflect this pattern, being almost exclusively restricted to the late spring to early autumn months. Hence, lesions erupting in winter are unlikely due to brown recluse spiders.[27]

Symptomatology and Pathophysiology

Envenomation by a recluse spider is known as loxoscelism. The resultant reaction can be placed into 4 categories: (1) unremarkable; (2) minor, self-healing symptoms; (3) dermonecrotic lesion; and (4) systemic loxoscelism. Categories 1 and 2 constitute

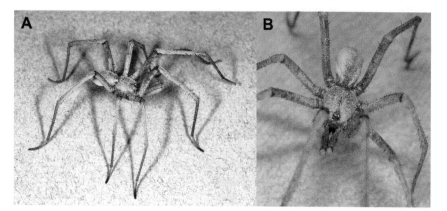

Fig. 5. Crevice weaver spider (genus *Kukulcania*) showing the overall body shape (*A*), and the head pattern that is mistaken for a violin shape (*B*). (Photos © R. Vetter.)

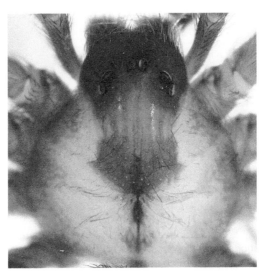

Fig. 6. Cephalothorax of brown recluse showing characteristic 6-eye pattern. (Photos © R. Vetter.)

about 90% of the reactions to *Loxosceles* spider bites.[28] Dermonecrotic lesions occur about 10% of the time and systemic loxoscelism is very rare, occurring in fewer than 1% of cases.[29] However, because medical reports of loxoscelism accentuate the more extreme, noteworthy manifestations of envenomation, with unremarkable bites being unheralded, the erroneous impression is generated that horrific wounds are the most common expression of the bite.

Mild bites
In the first 2 categories of mild bites, a small (5 mm) erythematous papule develops. It becomes firm before healing with localized pruritus. Supportive care is sufficient and the wound is self-limiting.

Dermonecrotic lesions
The timeline for development of a dermonecrotic wound is presented in **Box 1**. The following is synthesized from many review articles in the references. The pathophysiologic mechanism of recluse venom dermonecrosis is still being elucidated. It is

Table 1 Body location of *Loxosceles* spider bites	
Leg	34.8%
Arm	16.7%
Torso	12.0%
Hand	8.7%
Foot	5.2%
Face	1.5%
Neck	1.2%
Buttocks	1.0%
Shoulder	0.6%
Genitalia	0.6%

Box 1
Timetable for development of dermonecrotic recluse spider lesions

- Initial bite may be painless or just a slight pinprick sensation
- 2 to 6 hours: symptoms appear, there is mild to severe pain, pruritus, erythema
- 12 hours: a small blister may form, fluid is clear or reddened, not containing pus
- 12 to 24 hours: the lesion may turn from erythematous to violaceous around the bite; if the erythema persists then serious necrosis will not develop, if it turns violaceous then this is a sign that necrosis may ensue
- 36 hours: morbilliform eruptions may occur on the trunk, dissipating by the end of the first week
- 48 hours: if necrosis is impending, the hemorrhagic, ecchymotic discolorations coalesce, the wound either does not blanch with pressure or, if it blanches, capillary refill does not occur when pressure is released; the lesion has irregular borders, not circular or uniform in shape
- 3 to 4 days: necrosis begins
- 5 to 7 days: at the bite site, eschar formation occurs
- 7 to 14 days: central area of the wound becomes dark, slightly depressed, necrotic, and hardened; eschar sloughs
- 2 to 4 months: healing occurs

---

known that the venom component responsible for dermonecrosis is sphingomyelinase D (SMD). SMD destroys capillary endothelial tissue within the first 10 minutes after the bite, leading to the release of chemical mediators that kick off a cascade of physiologic events, including platelet aggregation to repair damaged endothelial tissue. SMD also causes erythrocyte lysis. Within 3 hours, there is an infiltration of polymorphonucleocytes (PMN) to the bite site and platelets cause microthrombi, decreasing circulation in the area and creating an ischemic zone. PMNs continue to accumulate for 48 hours. Within 6 hours, localized edema may occur. If a lesion becomes dermonecrotic, symptoms begin within 2 to 6 hours, including mild to severe pain, tenderness, pruritus, and transient erythema, which then gives way to induration. A lesion can develop at the bite site within hours to weeks and is almost always a singular focal event. Pain is related to ischemia, which is thought to be caused by either vasospasm or disruption of the neural myelin sheath. The bite site is tender on palpation. A bleb may form approximately 12 hours post bite, filled with clear or bloody fluid but not pus. By 12 to 24 hours, if the lesion turns from red to violaceous, impending severe necrosis is probable. A lesion that maintains its red color is a positive sign that necrosis will likely be mild or absent. The wound becomes ecchymotic, with irregular, asymmetric borders (symmetric borders are more indicative of Lyme disease). Damage can be intravascular (thrombosis) or extravascular (massive hemorrhaging into adjacent dermal and muscle tissue). By 36 hours, morbilliform eruptions may occur on the trunk, which dissipate by the end of the first week as ischemia abates. By 48 hours, if necrosis is impending, areas of hemorrhagic discoloration with uneven margins become confluent, no longer blanch on pressure, or do not refill after blanching. A bull's-eye wound may develop with a central bluish or violaceous cyanotic area, surrounded by white ischemia, then surrounded by erythema. On days 3 to 4 necrosis ensues, leading to eschar formation on days 5 to 7, although it could develop as early as a few hours to as late as a few weeks post bite. There is typically little swelling except in bites above the neck. Swelling in the face and periorbital area may be very pronounced, especially in children, and airway compromise is a concern. From days 7 to 14 the central area at the bite site becomes dark, depressed, necrotic, indurated, and devoid of sensation. Edges thicken and the eschar sloughs. Lesions are dry owing to compromised circulatory flow; they do not exude pus or serum. By days 14 to 21, debridement is recommended once the necrotic area is well defined and no longer spreading, and granulation is well under way. Debridement before this may increase healing time and increase disfiguration. Complete healing may require 2 to 4 months.

Dermonecrosis is exaggerated in obese victims because of the increased destruction of poorly vascularized adipose tissue. Wound extension may be gravitational because of another venom component, hyaluronidase, which digests the connective tissue matrix, allowing the venom to penetrate and spread more easily. Hyaluronidase is found in other venomous animals (eg, snakes)[30] as well as recluse spiders. In studies of recluse bites in America and Israel, delayed healing time was associated with increased age (older than 30 years or 10% increase for each decade of age), delayed treatment, and comorbid obesity, diabetes mellitus, and hypertension.[31,32] Although hemolysis is more commonly associated with systemic loxoscelism, evidence of mild hemolysis in patients in South America is reflected in elevated levels of bilirubin and lactate dehydrogenase.[33]

Systemic loxoscelism

In fewer than 1% of cases, recluse bites advance into a systemic syndrome that includes hemolytic anemia and acute kidney injury, most commonly in children. It may be fatal within 12 to 30 hours and, hence, represents a true emergency situation. Rapid recognition of this condition is critical. Symptoms can progress quickly, but if no hemolysis develops by 96 hours it is unlikely to occur. The venom is thought to act on metalloproteinases in the red blood cells, causing lysis. The volume of recluse venom is not capable of causing such extensive damage on its own, therefore the development of hemolytic anemia is thought to be triggered by mediators and other agents such as cytokines and interleukins. The local hemolysis spontaneously activates the complement system, leading to massive hemolysis and potential renal failure. Hemolytic anemia lasts from 4 to 7 days. The patient may experience chills, fever, malaise, nausea, vomiting, arthralgias, myalgias, and pruritus.[34] Petechial, scarlatiniform, or morbilliform eruptions on the trunk are common. Jaundice and scleral icterus develop as a result of increased bilirubin levels. Dark urine may be passed and oliguria can occur. Anemia is usually Coombs negative but can also be Coombs positive.[35] It is critical to perform blood work to monitor for hemoglobinemia, hemoglobinuria, thrombocytopenia, and acute kidney injury. Evidence points to direct nephrotoxicity of venom in addition to renal failure from hemoglobinuria[36] and rhabdomyolysis from local tissue damage.[37] Diagnosis is complicated by the ability of systemic loxoscelism to develop without dermonecrotic skin lesions, or before the lesions are physically evident. Additional systemic effects may include disseminated intravascular coagulation.

Treatment

Treatment of dermonecrosis

Although many remedies have been tried over the decades, most wounds respond well to simple RICE therapy (ie, Rest, Ice, Compression, Elevation). More recent data suggest that cold compresses are more helpful than ice, and support a neutral position rather than elevation.[38] Watchful waiting rather than early surgical debridement is advocated. Early debridement has been found to prolong healing times and result in greater disfiguration. Phillip Anderson, Missouri dermatologist and loxoscelism expert, stated that most recluse bites heal well on their own, and that debridement should only be used in severe necrotic events, and then only after the wound has stopped progressing.

In North America, in experimental situations antivenom has been administered with positive outcomes. Unfortunately, it is most effective if given within 24 hours of the bite,[39] but because most bite victims are initially unaware they have been bitten, they do not present for treatment until 48 hours post bite when envenomation symptoms become evident. Antivenom is more commonly used in South America for their native toxic species. One group of South American physicians advocates using antivenom after 24 hours, which, though less effective than if given earlier, still resulted in smaller lesions, faster healing times, and shorter hospital stays.[40] In other recent experimental work with rabbits, a topical tetracycline cream was effective in reducing the degree of necrosis when applied 6 hours after venom inoculation, whereby the mechanism of action is thought to be via inhibition of venom metalloproteinases.[41] (Oral tetracycline was not effective although the investigators state that low dosage might have been the cause, but cautioned that higher dosages had toxicity issues.) Attempts have been made to develop bioassays for confirming loxoscelism, with some success. Although there are no assays currently readily available in the clinical setting, an experimental enzyme-linked immunoassay test appears to be accurate, detecting sphingomyelinase down to 0.1 ng in wound assays.[42]

Outdated or ineffective treatments
Dapsone, an antileprosy drug and inhibitor of polymorphonucleocytes, was recommended for many years. However, dapsone may have significant clinical toxicity and can cause symptoms similar to those of recluse envenomation (hemolysis, drop in available hemoglobin). It also induces methemoglobinemia in patients with deficiency of glucose-6-phosphate dehydrogenase.[43] In one study, dapsone was found to increase scarring by 45%.[31] Given its toxicity profile and the possibility of worse outcome, this therapy is not recommended. Hyperbaric oxygen has been suggested, with some supporting studies, but additional studies have questioned its efficacy.[28] Other treatments such as electrical shock and nitroglycerin have some theoretical use and anecdotal success, but none of these treatments are of proven benefit[43] and may cause harm. Nitroglycerin was actually demonstrated to increase edema, inflammation, and creatine phosphokinase levels in rabbits injected with *Loxosceles* venom.[44] It will be difficult to provide evidence of efficacy for any treatment because of the unethical nature of withholding treatment from an envenomated patient, thereby creating a control group. In addition, recluse bites often heal spontaneously, further confounding experimental trials while emphasizing the necessity of control patients in experimental testing.

Treatment of systemic loxoscelism
Although systemic loxoscelism is dynamic and potentially life threatening, outcome is generally positive with corticosteroids, transfusions, and dialysis.[29,38] However, because death can occur rapidly, prompt action can be critical in patient survival.

Misdiagnosis
One area of great advancement in the last decade is the large body of information presented in attempts to shed light on the major problem of overdiagnosing skin lesions as spider bites.[20,43] In areas where recluse spider populations are rare or have never been documented, physicians frequently cite brown recluse spiders as the etiologic agents.[20,45–49] Although it is not impossible to have a recluse bite occur outside of

its endemic range,[50] this rare occurrence should not justify hundreds to thousands of bite diagnoses in nonendemic areas. Brown recluse diagnoses should be restricted to the endemic range of the spider unless a brown recluse, identified by an expert in arachnology, is captured in the act of biting.

Medical conditions that cause skin lesions similar to (or which have been previously misdiagnosed as) a brown recluse bite are presented in **Box 2**. Considering that outcome with recluse bites is generally positive, misdiagnosing another disease as loxoscelism may result in delayed or improper treatment of the true condition, allowing it to progress unmitigated. Missed diagnosis of conditions such as group A *Streptococcus*, lymphoma, cancer, and MRSA could lead to permanent disfigurement, loss of limbs, severe illness, or death. Misdiagnosis of pyoderma gangrenosum as loxoscelism could result in debridement, which increases injury caused by pathergy.[51] Lyme disease creates a bull's-eye wound, similar to loxoscelism, and occasionally manifests as a necrotic lesion.[52] Incorrect or delayed treatment of this condition may result in irreversible cardiac and neurologic problems. Despite widespread misconceptions in the general public and to some degree in the medical community, brown recluse bites do not result in amputations; limb loss is much more likely to be due to the misdiagnosis of necrotizing bacterial infection (such as group A *Streptococcus*) as loxoscelism.

YELLOW SAC SPIDERS

Yellow sac spiders are nonnative to North America and were rare on this continent before the mid-twentieth century, but are now found throughout most of America, commonly in homes. These spiders make small protective sacs in which they hide during the day, or lay their eggs and stay inside to guard them. Their sacs are often found in folds of curtains and in the tracks of sliding glass windows and doors.

In the 1970s, yellow sac spiders (genus *Cheiracanthium*) were implicated in mild necrotic skin lesions in North America and South Africa.[53,54] Although these reports were based on speculative or circumstantial evidence, yellow sac spiders were elevated to medical importance via repetitive citation in the medical literature rather than via evidence-based medicine.[55] A study including 20 verified yellow sac spider bites in North America and Australia and a review of 39 credible literature reports demonstrated that these spiders are unlikely sources of dermonecrosis.[55] Their bites are painful at inception, likened to a bee sting or splinter, and are associated with mild erythema, edema, and pruritus. Symptoms are self-limiting without major medical care. There were 2 reported cases of recurring pruritus over a 5-day period. No solid evidence implicates yellow sac spiders in causing necrotic skin lesions.

HOBO SPIDERS

The hobo spider (*Tegenaria agrestis*), a European immigrant, is found in the Pacific Northwest from British Columbia to Oregon, and east through Montana, Wyoming, Colorado, and northern Utah.[56] It is a generic brown spider, which looks like many other related spiders; to properly identify a hobo spider requires the skills of an arachnologist and the microscopic examination of its reproductive structures.[57] Hence, identifications by nonarachnologists are not definitive.

In the late 1980s, the hobo spider was implicated in dermonecrotic lesions in the Pacific Northwest, whereas before this time lesions were blamed on the nonexistent brown recluse spider.[58] Although the elevation of the hobo spider to medical importance was based predominantly on circumstantial evidence and was presented as a potential (but not definitive) etiologic factor,[59,60] this spider was readily accepted

Box 2
Medical conditions that result in necrotic skin lesions that could be or have been misdiagnosed as brown recluse spider bites

Infections

Atypical mycobacterial

Bacterial (*Staphylococcus*, *Streptococcus*, Lyme disease, cutaneous anthrax, syphilis, tularemia)

Deep fungal infections (sporotrichosis, aspergillosis)

Erythema gangrenosum

Environmental pathogens

Leishmaniasis

Viral (herpes simplex, herpes zoster)

Vascular Occlusive or Venous Disease

Venous status ulcers

Antiphospholipid-antibody syndrome

Livedoid vasculopathy

Small-vessel occlusive arterial disease

Necrotizing Vasculitis

Leukocytoclastic vasculitis

Polyarteritis nodosa

Takayasu arteritis

Wegener granulomatosis

Neoplastic Disease

Leukemia cutis

Lymphoma

Primary skin neoplasms (eg, basal cell carcinoma)

Topically Induced Conditions

Chemical and thermal burns

Poison ivy or poison oak

Factitious injury

Other Conditions

Arthropod bites

Calcific uremic arteriolopathy

Cryoglobulinemia

Diabetic ulcer

Langerhans cell histiocytosis

Lymphomatoid papulosis

Pemphigus vegetans

Pyoderma gangrenosum

Pressure ulcers

Radiotherapy

Septic embolism

Data from Swanson DL, Vetter RS. Bites of brown recluse spiders and suspected necrotic arachnidism. N Engl J Med 2005;352:700–7.

by the medical community as capable of causing severe dermonecrotic lesions. Subsequent work that attempted to duplicate the original research did not show a toxic effect when cleanly milked hobo spider venom was injected into the same strain of rabbits used in the original studies.[61] Hobo spider toxicity is currently being severely challenged.[61,62] Two arguments dispute the hobo spider being toxic. First, it is not considered dangerous in Europe, where the European scientific community has several centuries of experience with its fauna and flora. Second, this spider is large enough that fang puncture should hurt from mechanical piercing of skin; hence, if a hobo spider did bite, it would seem that more hobo spiders would be caught in the act of biting (ie, more than 2 verified bites in 80 years of the spider's existence in the Pacific Northwest).

OTHER SPIDERS

Many spiders are capable of piercing human skin and envenomating; however, most cause only minor, self-limited symptoms. Funnel weaving spiders (*Agelenopsis*, *Hololena*) have caused minor reactions in bite victims, with *Hololena* causing 4-hour periods of vomiting.[63,64] These mostly harmless North American spiders (family Agelenidae) should assuredly not be confused with the Sydney funnel web spider (family Hexathelidae), which is very distantly related and is highly toxic. Woodlouse spiders (*Dysdera crocata*) have long, imposing fangs that they brandish toward threats, but envenomation symptoms in verified bites subside within an hour. These spiders do occasionally invade homes.[65] Bites by green lynx spiders (*Peucetia*) leave only mild erythema,[66] but can spit venom 12 inches or so,[67] causing minor ocular injury.[68] Lynx spiders are common in gardens but not inside houses. Other spiders (orb weavers, wolf spiders) have been blamed for necrotic lesions, but this is not well substantiated and probably wrong, as subsequent documentation has demonstrated only minor effects.

Finally, one comment should be made about exotic spiders imported into North America, typically in shipments of bananas. The main danger does not come from the bite of an exotic and dangerous creature, but rather in having a biting spider misidentified as something extremely deadly when it is likely harmless. Subsequently, overzealous treatment could be worse than the potential envenomation effects. In several cases, large spiders with red facial hairs have been identified as the potentially dangerous and rarely deadly armed spider, *Phoneutria fera*, from South America.[69] Almost all of these spiders have actually been the harmless spider, *Cupiennius chiapanensis*. The armed spider lives in the Brazilian Amazon forest far from Central America and northwestern South America where bananas imported to North America originate, so it is unlikely to be a stowaway on these shipments.

MRSA AND OTHER BACTERIAL INFECTIONS

Possibly the most important advance in spider toxicology is the realization that many skin lesions that were attributed to spider bites were actually bacterial infections. Both physicians and patients made this misattribution.[70] In one nationwide study, 29% of 248 patients who presented with skin lesions and a chief complaint of spider bite actually had MRSA infections.[71] Another study showed that of 182 southern Californian patients seeking treatment for spider bites, only 3.8% had actual spider bites while 85.7% had infections.[72]

Although there are claims that spiders are vectors of bacteria, the substantiation of these speculative claims is not convincing, and studies show that this is unlikely.[73,74] Anderson[75] states that in consulting on approximately 1000 credible recluse spider bite cases in his career, not one was ever infected with bacteria or needed antibiotics. A study involving 750 verified spider bites (with a subsequent personal communication with the lead author) resulted in none causing confirmed or severe infection, and fewer than 1% developing mild or moderate symptoms of secondary infection (redness, swelling, pain, often delayed).[76] Spider venom is actually well known for its antibacterial properties and has been investigated for its potential use against resistant bacterial strains.[77,78] Although a spider bite leading to bacterial infection appears to be a feasible pathway of inoculation, evidence contradicts this association.

In some respects, the pendulum has swung from recluse bites to MRSA such that some physicians have misdiagnosed MRSA when it was actually loxoscelism.[79] However, misdiagnoses of loxoscelism still abound.

REPORTS FROM POISON CONTROL CENTERS

One final point should be made regarding spider envenomations. Authors of articles on spider bites often cite reports from poison control centers as reflections of spider-bite frequency for a specific geographic region. However, these data are generated from phone calls to the poison control center, mostly from the general public.[80] It is actually a tally of the perception of spider bites rather than a genuine report of cases diagnosed by medical personnel. Poison control data are reliable for unequivocal causative agents such as rattlesnake bite or aspirin overdose; however, for spider bites it is almost useless.[80] For example, reports from poison control centers of brown recluse spider bites in Florida and Georgia were very common in counties outside the native range of this spider where the spiders have never been documented.[47,48] Therefore, data from poison control centers must be interpreted with caution.

REFERENCES

1. Garb JE, Gonzalez A, Gillespie RG. The black widow spider genus *Latrodectus* (Araneae: Theridiidae): phylogeny, biogeography, and invasion history. Mol Phylogenet Evol 2004;31:1127–42.
2. Kaston BJ. Comparative biology of American black widow spiders. Trans San Diego Soc Nat Hist 1970;16:33–82.
3. Vetter RS, Vincent LS, Danielsen DW, et al. The prevalence of brown widow and black widow spiders (Araneae: Theridiidae) in urban southern California. J Med Entomol 2012;49:947–51.
4. Kirby-Smith HT. Black widow spider bite. Ann Surg 1942;115:249–57.
5. Clark RF, Wethern-Kestner S, Vance MV, et al. Clinical presentation and treatment of black widow spider envenomation: a review of 163 cases. Ann Emerg Med 1992;21:782–7.
6. Isbister GK, Fan HW. Spider bite. Lancet 2011;378:2039–47.
7. Wiener S. Red back spider bite in Australia: an analysis of 167 cases. Med J Aust 1961;2:44–9.
8. Offerman SR, Daubert GP, Clark RF. The treatment of black widow spider envenomation with antivenin *Latrodectus mactans*: a case series. Perm J 2011;15: 76–81.
9. Wolfe MD, Myers O, Caravati EM, et al. Black widow spider envenomation in pregnancy. J Matern Fetal Neonatal Med 2011;24:122–6.
10. Maretic Z, Lebez D. Genus *Latrodectus*. In: Maretic Z, Lebez D, editors. Araneism with special reference to Europe. Belgrade (Serbia): Nolit Publishing; 1979. p. 24–171.

11. Browning CC. Original investigations on spider bites in southern California. South Calif Pract 1901;16:291–300.
12. Suntorntham S, Roberts JR, Nilsen GJ. Dramatic clinical response to the delayed administration of black widow spider antivenin. Ann Emerg Med 1994;24:1198–9.
13. Graudins A, Padula M, Broady K, et al. Red-back spider (*Latrodectus hasselti*) antivenom prevents the toxicity of widow spider venoms. Ann Emerg Med 2001;37:154–60.
14. Müller GJ. Black and brown widow spider bites in South Africa: a series of 45 cases. S Afr Med J 1993;83:399–405.
15. Goddard J, Upshaw S, Held D, et al. Severe reaction from envenomation by the brown widow spider, *Latrodectus geometricus* (Araneae: Theridiidae). South Med J 2008;101:1269–70.
16. Cardosa JL, Brescovit AD, Haddad V Jr. Clinical aspects of human envenoming caused by *Latrodectus geometricus* (Theridiidae). J Venom Anim Toxins Incl Trop Dis 2003;9:418.
17. Kiriakos D, Núñez P, Parababire Y, et al. First case of human latrodectism in Venezuela. Rev Soc Bras Med Trop 2008;41:202–4.
18. Isbister GK, Gray MR. Effects of envenoming by comb-footed spiders of the genera *Steatoda* and *Achaearanea* (family Theridiidae: Araneae) in Australia. J Toxicol Clin Toxicol 2003;41:809–19.
19. Graudins A, Gunja N, Broady KW, et al. Clinical and in vitro evidence for the efficacy of Australian red-back spider (*Latrodectus hasselti*) antivenom in the treatment of envenomation by the cupboard spider (*Steatoda grossa*). Toxicon 2002; 40:767–75.
20. Vetter RS. Spiders of the genus *Loxosceles* (Araneae: Sicariidae): a review of biological, medical and psychological aspects regarding envenomations. J Arachnol 2008;36:150–63.
21. Saupe EE, Papes M, Selden PA, et al. Tracking a medically important arachnid: climate change, ecological niche modeling, and the brown recluse spider (*Loxosceles reclusa*). PLoS One 2011;6:17–31.
22. Vetter RS. Arachnids submitted as suspected brown recluse spiders (Araneae: Sicariidae): *Loxosceles* species are virtually restricted to their known distributions but are perceived to exist throughout the United States. J Med Entomol 2005;42: 512–21.
23. Vetter RS. Arachnids misidentified as brown recluse spiders by medical personnel and other authorities in North America. Toxicon 2009;54:545–7.
24. de Oliveira KC, de Andrade RM, Piazza RM, et al. Variations in *Loxosceles* spider venom composition and toxicity contribute to the severity of envenomation. Toxicon 2005;45:421–9.
25. de Olivera KC, Goncalves de Andrade RM, Giusti AL, et al. Sex-linked variation of *Loxosceles intermedia* spider venoms. Toxicon 1999;37:217–21.
26. Vetter RS. Seasonality of brown recluse spiders, *Loxosceles reclusa*, submitted by the general public: implications for physicians regarding loxoscelism diagnoses. Toxicon 2011;58:623–5.
27. Rader RK, Stoecker WV, Malters JM, et al. Seasonality of brown recluse populations is reflected by numbers of brown recluse envenomations. Toxicon 2012;60:1–3.
28. Tutrone WD, Green KM, Norris T, et al. Brown recluse spider envenomation: dermatologic application of hyperbaric oxygen therapy. J Drugs Dermatol 2005;4:424–8.
29. Anderson PC. Missouri brown recluse spider: a review and update. Mo Med 1998;95:318–22.

30. Meier J, Stocker KF. Biology and distribution of venomous snakes of medical importance and the composition of snake venoms. In: Meier J, White J, editors. Handbook of clinical toxicology of animal venoms and poisons. Boca Raton (FL): CRC Press; 1995. p. 367–412.

31. Mold JW, Thompson DM. Management of brown recluse spider bites in primary care. J Am Board Fam Pract 2004;17:347–52.

32. Dyachenko P, Ziv M, Rozenman D. Epidemiological and clinical manifestations of patients hospitalized with brown recluse spider bite. J Eur Acad Dermatol Venereol 2006;20:1121–5.

33. Malaque CM, Santoro ML, Cardoso JL, et al. Clinical picture and laboratorial evaluation in human loxoscelism. Toxicon 2011;58:664–71.

34. Hostetler MA, Dribben W, Wilson DB, et al. Sudden unexplained hemolysis occurring in an infant due to presumed *Loxosceles* envenomation. J Emerg Med 2003; 25:277–82.

35. Elbahlawan LM, Stidham GL, Bugnitz MC, et al. Severe systemic reaction to *Loxosceles reclusa* spider bites in a pediatric population. Pediatr Emerg Care 2005; 21:177–80.

36. Chaim OM, Sade YB, da Silveira RB, et al. Brown spider dermonecrotic toxin directly induces nephrotoxicity. Toxicol Appl Pharmacol 2006;211:64–77.

37. Franca FO, Barbaro KC, Abdulkader RC. Rhabdomyolysis in presumed viscerocutaneous loxoscelism: report of two cases. Trans R Soc Trop Med Hyg 2002;96: 287–90.

38. Wasserman GS, Lowry JA. *Loxosceles* spiders. In: Brent J, Wallace KL, Burkhart KK, et al, editors. Critical care toxicology: diagnosis and management of the critically poisoned patient. Philadelphia: Elsevier Mosby; 2005. p. 1195–203.

39. Rees R, Shack RB, Withers E, et al. Management of brown recluse spider bite. Plast Reconstr Surg 1981;68:768–73.

40. Pauli I, Puka J, Gubert IC, et al. The efficacy of antivenom in loxoscelism treatment. Toxicon 2006;48:123–37.

41. Paixão-Cavalcante D, van den Berg CW, Goncalves de Andrade RM, et al. Tetracycline protects against dermonecrosis induced by *Loxosceles* spider venom. J Invest Dermatol 2007;127:1410–8.

42. Gomez HF, Krywko DM, Stoecker WV. A new assay for the detection of *Loxosceles* species (brown recluse) spider venom. Ann Emerg Med 2002;39:469–74.

43. Swanson DL, Vetter RS. Bites of brown recluse spiders and suspected necrotic arachnidism. N Engl J Med 2005;352:700–7.

44. Lowry BP, Bradfield JF, Carroll RG, et al. A controlled trial of topical nitroglycerin in a New Zealand white rabbit model of brown recluse spider envenomation. Ann Emerg Med 2001;37:161–5.

45. Vetter RS, Cushing PE, Crawford RL, et al. Diagnoses of brown recluse spider bites (loxoscelism) greatly outnumber actual verifications of the spider in four western American states. Toxicon 2003;42:413–8.

46. Bennett RG, Vetter RS. An approach to spider bites: erroneous attribution of dermonecrotic lesions to brown recluse or hobo spider bites in Canada. Can Fam Physician 2004;50:1098–101.

47. Vetter RS, Edwards GB, James LF. Reports of envenomation by brown recluse spiders (Araneae: Sicariidae) outnumber verifications of *Loxosceles* spiders in Florida. J Med Entomol 2004;41:593–7.

48. Vetter RS, Hinkle NC, Ames LM. Distribution of the brown recluse spider (Araneae: Sicariidae) in Georgia with a comparison of poison center reports of envenomations. J Med Entomol 2009;46:15–20.

49. Frithsen IL, Vetter RS, Stocks IC. Reports of envenomation by brown recluse spiders exceed verified specimens of *Loxosceles* spiders in South Carolina. J Am Board Fam Med 2007;20:483–8.

50. Laack TA, Stead LG, Wolfe ME. Images in emergency medicine. Ann Emerg Med 2007;50:368–9.

51. Chow RK, Ho VC. Treatment of pyoderma gangrenosum. J Am Acad Dermatol 1996;34:1047–60.

52. Osterhout KC, Zaoutis T, Zorc JJ. Lyme disease masquerading as brown recluse spider bite. Ann Emerg Med 2002;39:558–61.

53. Spielman A, Levi HW. Probable envenomation by *Chiracanthium mildei*; a spider found in houses. Am J Trop Med Hyg 1970;19:729–32.

54. Newlands G, Martindale CB, Berson SD, et al. Cutaneous necrosis caused by the bite of *Chiracanthium* spiders. S Afr Med J 1980;57:171–3.

55. Vetter RS, Isbister GK, Bush SP, et al. Verified bites by *Cheiracanthium* spiders in the United States and Australia: where is the necrosis? Am J Trop Med Hyg 2006; 74:1043–8.

56. Vetter RS, Roe AH, Bennett RG, et al. Distribution of the medically-implicated hobo spider (Araneae: Agelenidae) and its harmless congener, *Tegenaria duellica*, in the United States and Canada. J Med Entomol 2004;40:159–64.

57. Vetter R, Antonelli A. How to identify (and misidentify) a hobo spider. Wash St Univ Coop Ext Pest Leaflet Series #116, 10 pp. Available at: http://pep.wsu.edu/pdf/PLS116_1.pdf. Accessed March 5, 2013.

58. Lee RV, Buker RS Jr, Petersen KM. North American loxoscelism: two presumptive cases from northern Montana. Rocky Mt Med J 1969;66:57–9.

59. Vest DK. Envenomation by *Tegenaria agrestis* (Walckenaer) spiders in rabbits. Toxicon 1987;25:221–4.

60. Vest DK. Necrotic arachnidism in the northwest United States and its probable relationship to *Tegenaria agrestis* (Walckenaer) spiders. Toxicon 1987;25:175–84.

61. Binford GJ. An analysis of geographic and intersexual chemical variation in venoms of the spider *Tegenaria agrestis* (Agelenidae). Toxicon 2001;39:955–68.

62. Vetter RS, Isbister GK. Do hobo spider bites cause dermonecrotic injuries? Ann Emerg Med 2004;44:605–7.

63. Vetter RS. Envenomation by an agelenid spider, *Agelenopsis aperta*, previously considered harmless. Ann Emerg Med 1998;32:739–41.

64. Vetter RS. Envenomation by spiders of the genus *Hololena* (Araneae: Agelenidae). Toxicon 2012;60:312–4.

65. Vetter RS, Isbister GK. Verified bites by the woodlouse spider, *Dysdera crocata*. Toxicon 2006;47:826–9.

66. Bush SP, Giem P, Vetter RS. Green lynx spider (*Peucetia viridans*) envenomation. Am J Emerg Med 2000;18:64–6.

67. Fink LS. Venom-spitting by the green lynx spider, *Peucetia viridans* (Araneae, Oxyopidae). J Arachnol 1984;12:372–3.

68. Tinkham ER. A poison-squirting spider. Bull U S Army Med Dep 1946;5:361–2.

69. Vetter RS, Hillebrecht S. On distinguishing two often-misidentified genera (*Cupiennius, Phoneutria*) (Araneae: Ctenidae) of large spiders found in Central and South American cargo shipments. Amer Entomol 2008;54:82–7.

70. Dominguez TJ. It's not a spider bite, it's community-acquired methicillin-resistant *Staphylococcus aureus*. J Am Board Fam Pract 2004;17:220–6.

71. Moran GJ, Krishnadasan A, Gorwitz RJ, et al. Methicillin-resistant *S. aureus* infections among patients in emergency rooms. N Engl J Med 2006;355: 666–74.

72. Suchard JR. "Spider bite" lesions are usually diagnosed as skin and soft-tissue infections. J Emerg Med 2011;41:473–81.
73. Baxtrom C, Mongkolpradit T, Kasimos JN, et al. Common house spiders are not likely vectors of community-acquired methicillin-resistant *Staphylococcus aureus* infections. J Med Entomol 2006;43:962–5.
74. Gaver-Wainwright MM, Zack RS, Foradori MJ, et al. Misdiagnosis of spider bites: bacterial associates, mechanical pathogen transfer, and hemolytic potential of venom from the hobo spider, *Tegenaria agrestis* (Araneae: Agelenidae). J Med Entomol 2011;48:382–8.
75. Anderson PC. Spider bites in the United States. Dermatol Clin 1997;15:307–11.
76. Isbister GK, Gray MR. A prospective study of 750 definite spider bites, with expert spider identification. QJM 2002;95:723–31.
77. Yan L, Adams ME. Lycotoxins, antimicrobial peptides from venom of the wolf spider *Lycosa carolinensis*. J Biol Chem 1998;273:2059–66.
78. Benli M, Yigit N. Antibacterial activity of venom from funnel web spider *Agelena labyrinthica* (Araneae: Agelenidae). J Venom Anim Toxins Incl Trop Dis 2008;14: 641–50.
79. Rogers KM, Klotz CR, Jack M, et al. Systemic loxoscelism in the age of community-acquired methicillin-resistant *Staphylococcus aureus*. Ann Emerg Med 2011;57:138–40.
80. Vetter RS, Furbee RB. Caveats in interpreting poison control centre data for spider bites in epidemiology studies. Public Health 2006;120:179–81.

Review of Human Rabies Prophylaxis and Treatment

Kyle A. Weant, PharmD, BCPS[a],*, Stephanie N. Baker, PharmD, BCPS[b,c]

KEYWORDS

- Rabies • Rabies virus • Rabies vaccine • Lyssavirus
- Human rabies immune globulin • Antivirals • Immunizations • Human rabies

KEY POINTS

- Rabies is an acute, progressive encephalitis caused by a mammalian virus and carries with it an associated mortality of close to 100%.
- When used appropriately, postexposure prophylaxis after exposure to the rabies virus is universally effective.
- Postexposure prophylaxis involves adequate wound care, infiltration of rabies immune globulin, and vaccine administration.
- The treatment of human rabies infection is largely palliative, because no therapy has been shown to be effective.

INTRODUCTION

Rabies is an acute, progressive encephalitis caused by a group of RNA viruses that use mammals as reservoirs.[1,2] Although worldwide, rabies results in the deaths of more than 55,000 people annually, rabies is uncommon in developed nations.[3–8] One of the factors that makes this virus so unique is its associated mortality of close to 100% when prophylactic measures are not undertaken in an appropriate time frame. Fewer than 2 deaths are reported each year in the United States, down from more than 100 per year at the beginning of the twentieth century.[9] In addition to significant improvements in animal control, this decrease is in large part a result of the availability of postexposure prophylaxis, which has been proved to be almost 100%

Disclosures: None.
Conflict of Interest: None.
[a] North Carolina Public Health Preparedness and Response, North Carolina Department of Health and Human Services, 100 East Six Forks Road, Suite 150, Raleigh, NC 27699-1900, USA; [b] Department of Pharmacy Services, UK Health Care, 800 Rose Street, H110, Lexington, KY 40536-0293, USA; [c] Department of Pharmacy Practice and Science, University of Kentucky College of Pharmacy, 800 Rose Street, H110, Lexington, KY 40536, USA
* Corresponding author.
E-mail address: kaw9600@alumni.unc.edu

Crit Care Nurs Clin N Am 25 (2013) 225–242
http://dx.doi.org/10.1016/j.ccell.2013.02.001
0899-5885/13/$ – see front matter © 2013 Elsevier Inc. All rights reserved.

effective when used appropriately. However, this decrease in mortality comes at a significant cost to the health care system through its requisite time intensity and investment of substantial monetary resources; postexposure prophylaxis is complex, lengthy, and costly.[10] The estimated public health costs associated with disease prevention, detection, and control exceed $300 million in the United States annually.[11] Therefore, because of the high risk of mortality and the large financial investment that the US health care system has put toward the protection of the public from this devastating virus, it is imperative that all health care practitioners become familiar with the appropriate prevention of this disease and are prepared to implement aggressive treatment should the need arise.

TRANSMISSION

The neurotropic viruses that cause rabies are RNA viruses with multiple genotypes of the family Rhabdoviridae and genus *Lyssavirus*.[2,12–14] All rabies strains in North America are of genotype 1. Lyssaviruses move through the peripheral nervous system to their target, the central nervous system (CNS), where replication occurs.[15] From the brain, the virus travels to other organs or glands, such as the salivary glands, where it is excreted abundantly. This excretion of the virus may precede, be simultaneous, or occur after the development of clinical signs and symptoms. The rabies virus is not viable outside the host and can be inactivated by sunlight, heat, and desiccation.[16] As a result, exposure must occur when there is penetration of the skin by teeth or, less commonly, through direct transdermal or mucosal contact. The most common and important route of transmission is through infected saliva after a bite.[17]

All mammals are susceptible and can transmit the rabies virus, but the primary reservoir worldwide is carnivorous mammals, including dogs and foxes, as well as bats.[18] In North America, raccoons and skunks also serve as important reservoirs. Technically, all mammals are susceptible to infection, but there is great interspecies variability with regards to being important reservoirs. Dogs are the major reservoir and vector worldwide for this virus, causing most human deaths each year.[19] However, canine vaccination programs and control of stray animals have greatly reduced the cases of domestic animal rabies in the United States, with dog rabies declining 90% in the last decade.[18,20] Subsequently, wild animals are the most important potential source of infection for both humans and domestic animals in the United States. In 2011, wild animals represented 91.8% of the rabid animals reported.[21] In the same year, most cases of rabies occurred among raccoons (32.8%), skunks (27%), bats (22.9%), and foxes (7.1%). Since 2002, 87.5% of naturally acquired, indigenous human rabies cases in the United States have resulted from variants of rabies viruses associated with bats.[18,21]

In the last 50 years, few nonbite exposures have been documented in humans.[22] Only 51 cases have been described in the literature as not being transmitted as the result of animal bites.[23–25] Most of the reported cases were caused by inadequately inactivated vaccine. Potential does exists for infection to occur through inhalation of the virus, although this may be possible only in research settings during the manipulation of tissue, because there is 1 documented case. Inhalation transmission can also occur in caves where bat density is high and minimal ventilation exists, as documented by 2 cases in Texas for which other plausible explanations exist.[22,26] Infrequently, human-to-human transmission has been reported. In 2004, 4 transplant recipients in the United States became infected from an infected organ donor, all resulting in the deaths of the organ recipients.[18,27,28] There is only 1 report of a human with encephalitic rabies biting another human.[29] In this case, the individual received postexposure prophylaxis and did not develop the disease. Although human-to-human transmission is possible, no cases have been documented among health care workers. Standard barrier precautions should be used whenever caring for an infected patient to minimize any risk of transmission that may exist.

INFECTION
Clinical Presentation

Clinical rabies can have a wide variety of presentations and essentially all are possible for the most part regardless of the species. Typical signs and symptoms can include low-grade fever, lack of appetite, paresthesias, ataxia, anxiety, altered mentation, paralysis, coma, and death. Specific symptoms such as hydrophobia and aerophobia are believed to be limited to human beings.[30] These phobias may present as pharyngeal and laryngeal spasms when infected patients attempt to drink water (hydrophobia) or feel a breeze (aerophobia). In humans, some laboratory abnormalities have been noted in the limited cases available, including abnormal cerebrospinal fluid results in 87% of patients.[29]

Incubation

Human rabies typically manifests in 5 stages: incubation period, prodrome, acute neurologic phase, coma, and death. The duration of the incubation period ranges from a few days to several years, but in about 60% of cases it is 1 to 3 months.[12,16] The virus binds to nicotinic receptors on the surface of muscle fibers, replicates slowly within muscle, and then travels into nerve tissue through neuromuscular junctions.[12,16,27] The variation in incubation periods may be associated with the time required to replicate within muscle tissue and transverse into neuronal axons. Deep lacerations or bites occurring on the head and neck, in which the virus is directly inoculated into nerve tissue, are generally associated with shorter incubation periods.

Prodrome

The prodromal stage begins once the virus has traveled from the peripheral nervous system to the CNS, resulting in symptoms such as fever, headache, malaise, irritability, nausea, and vomiting.[31] Paresthesias, pain, and pruritus may arise locally at the site of viral entry.[12,16] The prodrome generally lasts 2 to 10 days. Progression from the prodromal stage to the acute neurologic phase is characterized by neurologic dysfunction. At this point, the virus begins replicating within the CNS and then moves out to other organs and glands.[31] These organs and glands may include not only the salivary glands but the myocardium as well.[32]

Acute Neurologic Phase

The acute neurologic phase lasts up to a week and can manifest as encephalitic or paralytic rabies. Encephalitic rabies is the most common presentation, accounting for 80% of the documented cases.[33] These symptoms include hyperexcitability, hyperactivity, hallucinations, excessive salivation, hydrophobia, and aerophobia.[12,31] Once the encephalitic form of rabies presents, patient death typically follows within 5 days.[12] Paralytic rabies presents differently, usually starting with paralysis of the limb initially exposed to the virus. This paralysis can progress to quadriplegia symmetrically or asymmetrically, and also leads to urinary and fecal incontinence. Death can occur secondary to the development of diaphragmatic and bulbar paralysis within a few weeks.[16]

Coma

Coma occurs in the late stages of clinical progression in both the encephalitic and paralytic forms and is associated with multiorgan failure and autonomic instability.[34] Coma is secondary to functional damage in the hypothalamus and brain stem territories, resulting in adverse cardiac and respiratory consequences.[35] It can last anywhere between 5 and 14 days.

Death

The causes of death can be multifactorial in this infection, with cardiac and respiratory disorders being common. Cardiac disorders occur in almost all cases, including sinus tachycardia, heart failure, and hypotension, with the cause of death being related to cardiac and circulatory insufficiency.[16] Cardiac arrhythmias are also possible, including wandering atrial/nodal pacemaker, sinus bradycardia, and supraventricular or ventricular ectopic beats.[36,37] Common respiratory complications include hyperventilation, hypoxemia, respiratory depression, and atelectasis.[36] In addition, hematemesis occurs in approximately 30% to 60% of patients during the last few hours before death.[12] An overview of these 5 stages is presented in **Table 1**.

Diagnosis

The diagnosis of rabies should be based on both suggestive clinical signs and symptoms and objective test results. For patients presenting with possible encephalitic rabies, the differential diagnosis should also include tetanus, diphtheria, botulism, and substance abuse.[12,16] Conditions that should be included in the differential diagnosis when considering a patient presenting with possible paralytic rabies include Guillain Barré syndrome, Japanese encephalitis, cerebral malaria, and the West Nile virus. Radiologic imaging, such as magnetic resonance imaging, may provide additional clues to the accurate diagnosis.[12]

Because of the progressive nature of this disease and its self-isolation within the CNS, laboratory test sensitivities can have significant variability concerning the diagnosis of rabies.[12,16] Because the virus is present in saliva only after replication in the CNS and may not spread to all salivary glands, or is secreted only intermittently, the

Table 1
Stages of human rabies infection

Stage	Approximate Duration	Explanation
Incubation	1–3 mo	Time required for virus replication and movement into neural tissue
Prodrome	2–10 d	Arrival of the virus in the CNS. Symptoms include fever, headache, malaise, irritability, nausea, and vomiting
Acute neurologic phase	1 wk	Phase can manifest as encephalitic or paralytic rabies. Symptoms include hyperexcitability, hyperactivity, hallucinations, excessive salivation, hydrophobia, and aerophobia
Coma	5–14 d	The result of brain stem and hypothalamic damage. Associated with multiorgan failure and autonomic instability
Death	Variable	The cumulative impact of cardiac, respiratory, and organ failure from other stages, leading to an increased risk of cardiac arrhythmias and respiratory depression

definitive diagnosis of rabies lies in brain tissue assessment. A test of brain tissue provides a clear positive or negative diagnosis regarding exposure to the rabies virus.[30] Although this postmortem approach to diagnosis is effective in animals, surrogate markers must be used during antemortem testing in suspected human cases.[7] Possible specimens include serum, cerebrospinal fluid, saliva, and skin from highly innervated locations. The appearance of antibodies to specific rabies antigens, or rabies viral RNA, is diagnostic in a patients with no history of previous vaccination and presenting with suggestive clinical symptoms. The production of antibodies does not occur in all individuals and generally takes 7 to 10 days after the onset of symptoms, further complicating the diagnosis. The Centers for Disease Control and Prevention (CDC) or state health officials should be contacted to help aid in diagnosis.

Although the isolation of a clear negative diagnosis of rabies allows for the exploration of other causes of the neurologic sequelae, isolating a positive rabies diagnosis yields minimal benefit for the patient. Although it does result in the cessation of the search for competing causes, because no real treatment options exist for this disease, the care of the patient does not necessarily improve. However, establishing the correct diagnosis is important from a public health perspective, because it allows officials to better identify any risk to the public health and aids in the development of mitigation strategies.

VACCINES

Available rabies vaccines are inactivated virus vaccines that induce an active immune response, resulting in the production of virus neutralizing antibodies. This production is typically delayed 7 to 10 days, although the antibodies generally persist for several years.[38,39] Three cell-culture rabies vaccines are licensed in the United States: human diploid cell vaccine (Imovax Rabies, Sanofi Pasteur, Swiftwater, PA, USA), purified chick embryo cell vaccine (RabAvert, Novartis Vaccines and Diagnostics, Emeryville, CA, USA), and rabies vaccine adsorbed (Bioport Corporation, Lansing, MI, USA).[17] However, only Imovax and RabAvert are available for use in the United States. Both Imovax and RabAvert are preservative free and should be administered immediately after reconstitution.[38,39] They should be stored protected from light at 2°C to 8°C and should not be frozen. For both vaccines, the total volume of 1 dose is 1 mL (a full 1.0-mL intramuscular (IM) dose is used for both preexposure and postexposure prophylaxis regimens) and should be administered IM into the deltoid region. In young children and infants, the vaccines may be injected into the anterolateral area of the thigh, if necessary. Gluteal administration is not recommended, because this may result in lower neutralizing antibody titers and may damage the sciatic nerve.[40] The vaccines should not be administered subcutaneously, intradermally, or intravascularly. In an attempt to reduce costs in developing countries, some have experimented with the use of intradermal versus IM injections.[41] However, this route is not approved in the United States and should not be attempted until further data are available. The US Food and Drug Administration (FDA) requires all US licensed rabies vaccines for human use to have a potency of each dose equal to, or greater than, the World Health Organization's recommended standard of 2.5 IU per 1.0 mL of vaccine.[17,42] A vaccination series is initiated and completed usually with 1 product; however, switching to another product may be considered if adverse effects prove intolerable.[43,44] RabAvert should be avoided in patients with severe egg allergies because the vaccine is prepared with chick embryos and may contain a small amount of egg protein. No comparative clinical trials exist to ascertain a superiority of 1 vaccine product compared with another.

Adverse Effects

Adverse effects commonly associated with the use of either rabies vaccine include local injection site reactions such as erythema, itching, and swelling and systemic reactions such as headache, nausea, abdominal pain, muscle aches, dizziness, and fever. Studies regarding adverse events have shown that these local reactions can occur in close to 90% of patients.[45–47] Injection site pain is the most common local reaction, occurring in 20% to 70% of patients in some studies.[48,49] Systemic hypersensitivity reactions have been reported in 6% of persons receiving booster vaccinations, with half of these occurring 6 to 14 days after injection.[50] Rare, neurologic disorders have been reported; however, these side effects are limited to case reports.[51,52] Because they are derivatives of human blood, they do have a risk of transmitting viral diseases and a theoretic risk for transmitting Creutzfeldt-Jakob disease (CJD). The occurrence of adverse effects should not interrupt the vaccination schedule and prophylaxis should not be discontinued after the development of local, or tolerable, signs and symptoms.[31]

IMMUNE GLOBULIN

The production of antibodies, and thus development of active immunity, after the administration of the rabies vaccine is delayed 7 to 10 days. The administration of virus neutralizing antibodies for passive immunity is necessary in the setting of postexposure prophylaxis.[43] Human rabies immune globulin (HRIG) is indicated only for those who have not previously been vaccinated and should be administered concomitantly with the vaccine, preferably with the first dose. Use of HRIG provides a rapid, passive immunity that persists for a short period.[53] After IM injection, antibodies are present in the serum within 24 hours and persists for approximately 21 days.[54,55] Studies have shown that administration of HRIG in conjunction with the rabies vaccine is more effective than either alone.[56]

Two antirabies immune globulin formulations are licensed and available for use in the United States: HyperRab S/D (Talecris Biotherapeutics, Research Triangle Park, NC, USA) and Imogam Rabies-HT (Sanofi Pasteur, Swiftwater, PA, USA).[54,55] Both products are preservative-free immunoglobulin preparations obtained from pooled plasma of human donors hyperimmunized with the rabies vaccine. The minimal potency of each is 150 IU/mL, and both products are available in 2-mL (300-IU) and 10-mL (1500-IU) vials, which should remain refrigerated (2–8°C) and should not be frozen. The recommended dose of HRIG is 20 IU/kg.[54,55] HRIG contains no preservative and should be used or discarded immediately. In all postexposure prophylaxis regimens, except for persons previously vaccinated, HRIG should be administered concurrently with the first dose of vaccine. HRIG should not be administered more than 7 days after the rabies vaccine, because it may interfere with active immune response and antibody production. If there exists a bite wound or site of infection, as much of the dose as is feasible should be injected around the wound.[54,55] Any remainder of the dose is administered IM, in the deltoid or quadriceps (at a location other than that used for vaccine inoculation to minimize the potential for interference).[14] Virus neutralization has been shown to be most effective when HRIG was injected directly around the wound, whereas only distant injection significantly increased the risk of viral infection of the CNS.[57] If no wound is visible, then the entire dose should be administered in the deltoid or quadriceps at a site other than the vaccine. This procedure may require multiple injections depending on the weight-based dose necessary for each patient. Rabies vaccine and HRIG should never be mixed in the same syringe.

The use of current formulations of HRIG is not associated with the acquisition of disease.[14] However, these formulations are blood products and therefore they may contain antibodies to other agents and thus inhibit immune responses to noninactivated viral vaccines. The administration of live vaccines, such as measles, mumps, rubella, and varicella, should be delayed for at least 3 to 4 months after postexposure prophylaxis to allow the degradation of HRIG.[58,59] If the interval is shorter, additional vaccination with the appropriate agent may be necessary, unless deemed not necessary through laboratory analysis of antibodies. As with the rabies vaccine, HRIG also carries with it the potential for the transmission of viral diseases and CJD.

One study exploring the adverse events associated with HRIG found that local reactions occurred in 75% to 100% of patients, depending on which formulation was used, and systemic reactions were reported in 75% to 81% of patients, with headache being the most common reaction.[60] No serious adverse events, including immediate hypersensitivity reactions or immune complex–like diseases were reported. In general, local reactions were more common with Imogam and systemic reactions were more common with HyperRab. In addition, those persons with IgA deficiency have an increased potential for developing antibodies to IgA and could have anaphylactic reactions.[54,55]

PREEXPOSURE PROPHYLAXIS

The concept of preexposure prophylaxis for rabies is used for several reasons. It provides some level of protection for those who may be at a high or continuous risk of contracting the virus and it provides protection to those persons who are at risk for an unrecognized exposure to rabies.[17] Although preexposure vaccination does not eliminate the need for additional vaccine administrations after exposure, it does simplify the management of patients by alleviating the need for HRIG and decreasing the total number of doses of vaccine necessary. Preexposure vaccination also provides additional protection for those individuals that might not have ready access to appropriate vaccines, or HRIG, immediately after an exposure, allowing them time to obtain the optimal medical care.[14]

Preexposure vaccination should be offered to groups who are at high and continuous risk for infection, such as veterinarians and their staff, animal handlers, rabies researchers, and certain laboratory workers. Preexposure vaccination should also be considered for persons whose activities bring them into frequent contact with the rabies virus or potentially rabid bats, raccoons, skunks, cats, dogs, or other species at risk for having rabies.

Some international travelers might be candidates for preexposure vaccination if they are likely to come in contact with animals in areas where dog or other animal rabies is enzootic and immediate access to appropriate medical care, including rabies vaccine and immune globulin, might be limited. Routine preexposure prophylaxis for the general US population, or routine travelers to areas where rabies is not enzootic, is not recommended.[61,62] Rabies vaccination is not warranted for most routine international travel because it does not provide a substantial risk, with only 0.4% experiencing an animal bite per month's stay in a rabies-endemic country.[61,63] In the last decade, 22 cases of rabies have been reported in travelers, 66% of whom did not receive correct postexposure prophylaxis.[64,65] Guidelines related to travel are available from the CDC to further delineate those at higher risk (http://www.cdc.gov/travel/diseases/rabies.htm). The CDC divides those groups at risk into 4 different categories (**Table 2**).[17] Preexposure prophylaxis is recommended for those populations who fall into the continuous, frequent, and infrequent groups. However, it is not

Table 2
Risk categories for preexposure prophylaxis

Risk Category	Population Included
Continuous	Rabies research laboratory works; rabies biologics production workers
Frequent	Rabies diagnostic laboratory workers, cavers, veterinarians and staff, and animal-control and wildlife workers in areas where rabies is enzootic. All persons who frequently handle bats
Infrequent	Veterinarians and animal-control staff working with terrestrial animals in areas where rabies is uncommon to rare. Veterinary students. Travelers visiting areas where rabies is enzootic and immediate access to appropriate medical care including biologics is limited
Rare	Population-at-large in the United States

recommended for those who fall into the rare group. After determining the appropriate group needing preexposure prophylaxis, it should be administered according to the following schedule: 3 1.0-mL injections of Imovax or RabAvert should be administered by IM injection in the deltoid area, 1 injection per day on days 0, 7, and 21 (or 28).[17]

Rabies virus neutralizing antibody levels do indicate the immune status to rabies; however, their correlation with infection susceptibility is unclear.[17] Based on the Advisory Committee for Immunization Practices (ACIP) recommendations, periodic measuring of rabies virus neutralizing antibody levels should be performed based on an individual's risk for exposure.[17] Individuals at a continuous risk should undergo titer testing every 6 months, and those who fall into the frequent-risk category for rabies exposure should have their titers measured every 2 years. Those at rare risk for exposure to rabies are not recommended to undergo serologic testing or to receive booster doses. A single booster dose of the vaccine should be given to individuals in the continuous-risk and frequent-risk categories when their titer levels are less than 0.5 IU/mL or if their titer fails to completely neutralize virus at a 1:5 serum dilution.

If an individual who has received preexposure prophylaxis is exposed to rabies, local wound care remains a critical part of postexposure prophylaxis. After appropriate wound management, these persons should receive 2 IM doses (1.0 mL each in the deltoid) of the vaccine, 1 immediately and 1 3 days later. Administration of HRIG is unnecessary and should not be administered because it may inhibit the relative strength or rapidity of an expected anamnestic response.[66] For previously vaccinated persons who are exposed to rabies, attempting to ascertain the rabies virus neutralizing antibody titer for decision making about prophylaxis is inappropriate because it delays care. In addition, the correlation of titers and infectious risk is unknown.

POSTEXPOSURE PROPHYLAXIS

It is estimated that approximately 23,000 people receive postexposure prophylaxis in the United States on an annual basis.[67,68] To maximize efficacy, minimize adverse effects, and limit health care expenditures, it is imperative to accurately differentiate a possible rabies exposure from a routine animal bite. The administration of rabies postexposure prophylaxis is urgent; however, it is not a medical emergency. Nevertheless, appropriate prophylaxis should not be delayed unnecessarily. The risks of inadequate treatment outweigh the risks associated with unnecessary treatment and so practitioners should err on the side of treatment in uncertain situations.[51,69]

The type of animal exposure should be classified as bite versus nonbite. The most likely mode of transmission occurs when a known rabid animal bites a potential host. A nonbite scenario can be created when rabid animal saliva is introduced into fresh, open cuts on the skin or onto mucous membranes, resulting in a nonbite transmission.[17] Indirect contact activities such as petting or handling an animal and contact with blood or saliva on intact skin does not constitute an exposure. Unprovoked animal attacks are more likely than provoked attacks to indicate that an animal may be infected.[17] Bites sustained while attempting to feed or handle an apparently healthy animal should generally be regarded as provoked. When assessing the risk of rabies transmission, the following should be considered: type of exposure; epidemiology of animal rabies in the area where the contact occurred and species of animal involved; circumstances of the exposure incident; availability of the exposing animal for observation or rabies testing.

Bat exposures warrant exceptional considerations when classifying as bite or nonbite exposures. The most common rabies virus variants responsible for human rabies in the United States are bat related, and all exposures require evaluation.[17] A bite from a rabid bat may go unnoticed by the potential host, and therefore, postexposure prophylaxis is indicated, regardless of a clear route of transmission. With any wild animal bite, if the animal is unavailable for testing, postexposure prophylaxis should be considered.

Both national and international organizations recommend that postexposure prophylaxis in a previously unvaccinated patient should be composed of wound care, infiltration of rabies immune globulin, and vaccine administration.[43,70] When a bite wound is evident, it should be promptly and thoroughly cleansed with soap and water.[57,71] Cleansing has been shown to be effective in reducing rabies transmission. The use of virucidal antiseptics such as povidone iodine and ethanol is advocated for initial wound treatment. Topical antibiotics may also be considered, depending on wound severity. In addition, closure of bite or scratch wounds should be avoided if possible.[72]

With the exception of persons who have previously received complete preexposure or postexposure vaccination regimens, the combination of HRIG and rabies vaccine is recommended after the determination of a possible rabies exposure, regardless of the interval between exposure and initiation of prophylaxis. Those who have previously received complete preexposure or postexposure vaccine regimens should receive only the vaccine. HRIG is administered only once to previously unvaccinated persons to provide immediate coverage until the patient responds to the vaccine by producing their own antibodies.[17] If HRIG is not administered when vaccination was begun, it can be administered up to and including day 7 of the prophylaxis series.[73] Beyond the seventh day, HRIG is not indicated, because an antibody response to cell-culture vaccine is presumed to have occurred. Because HRIG can partially suppress active production of antibody, the dose administered should not exceed the recommended dose.[74] The recommended dose of HRIG is 20 IU/kg (0.133 mL/kg) of total body weight. This formula is applicable to all age and weight groups, including children. If anatomically feasible, the full dose of HRIG should be thoroughly infiltrated in the area around and into the wounds. Any remaining volume should be injected IM at a site distant from vaccine administration. This recommendation for HRIG administration is based on reports of rare failures of postexposure prophylaxis when less than the full amount of HRIG was infiltrated at the exposure sites.[75] HRIG should never be administered in the same syringe or in the same anatomic site as the first vaccine dose. However, subsequent doses of vaccine in the 4-dose series can be administered in the same anatomic location where the HRIG was administered.

Either of the rabies vaccines available for use in the United States can be administered in conjunction with HRIG at the beginning of postexposure prophylaxis. Patients who have not been previously vaccinated, with a pre- or postexposure prophylaxis regimen should receive 4 1-mL doses of either rabies vaccine.[14,17] This strategy reflects a recent amendment of the ACIP recommendations that decreases the number of rabies vaccine doses required for postexposure prophylaxis from 5 to 4 based on current evidence and thus eliminates the vaccination requirement on day 28.[34] This decision was supported by a review of the literature that showed that in 1000 human individuals, virus neutralizing antibodies to rabies were present in all patients at 2 weeks.[76] Also, in an analysis of 1762 patients exposed to rabies, 25% of whom received less than 5 doses of the vaccine, no cases of human rabies were documented.[34] In addition to being clinically equivalent, this change from a 5-dose to a 4-dose schedule is estimated to save the US health care system $16.6 million.[34] However, patients who are immunosuppressed should still receive a 5-dose series of the vaccine on days 0, 3, 7, 14, and 28. The first dose of the 4-dose or 5-dose course should be administered as soon as possible after exposure. This date is then considered day 0 of the postexposure prophylaxis series. Additional doses should then be administered on days 3, 7, 14 (and 28 if immunosuppressed) after the first vaccination. Subsequent doses should ideally be obtained at a location other than the emergency department, such as a local health department or primary care office, if possible.

Cases of human rabies in the United States in which there is no history of contact with a rabid animal are common, and molecular analysis has shown that most of these cases are associated with bat rabies viruses.[26] Although rabies is not commonly reported in free-ranging bats and is diagnosed in less than 6% of bats submitted for public health evaluation, exposure to bats where any possibility of a bite exists constitutes a need for postexposure prophylaxis.[21] This exposure includes situations in which persons were in the same room as a bat and might have been unaware that a bite or direct contact had occurred.[43] Examples include a sleeping person awakening to find a bat in the room or a bat witnessed in the room with an unattended child, a person with intellectual disability, or an intoxicated person. If the bat is available for testing and the results are negative, postexposure prophylaxis may be discontinued. However, as more commonly is the case, prophylaxis should begin if the bat is unavailable for examination.[43]

According to experimental data and epidemiologic observations, some domestic species may be observed for signs of rabies. If a healthy dog or cat bites a human and rabies infection is suspected, the animal may be observed for 10 days.[77] If the animal remains healthy, the patient does not need postexposure prophylaxis. If the animal becomes ill with symptoms consistent with rabies, it should be killed and brain tissue should be tested for the virus. If the infection is confirmed within 24 to 48 hours after the animal is killed, there is adequate time to begin prophylaxis. If the animal is unknown to the human, such as a stray or wild animal, or displays symptoms, postexposure prophylaxis should begin on presentation. If postexposure prophylaxis has been initiated and appropriate laboratory diagnostic testing indicates that the exposing animal was not rabid, postexposure prophylaxis can be discontinued.[17]

Although postexposure prophylaxis recommendations are not always followed, no failures have been documented since current biologics have been licensed.[17] Most deaths are associated with humans who are unaware that they were bitten and thus have not obtained postexposure prophylaxis.[26] Postexposure prophylaxis should be instituted whenever exposure is suspected, and it is warranted regardless of the interval between exposure and presentation. Delays in initiating prophylaxis are associated with treatment failure.[78] Incubation periods can be between 2 weeks and 1 year.[5–7,79] The extent of delay that renders postexposure prophylaxis ineffective is not known.[80]

Adherence to the vaccination schedule is important, and although delays of a few days for individual doses may have a negligible effect, the impact of longer lapses of weeks or more is unclear.[14] For minor deviations from the immunization schedule, vaccination can be resumed where it was left off and the same interval should be maintained between doses. When substantial deviations from the schedule occur, immune status should be assessed by performing serologic testing 7 to 14 days after administration of the final dose in the series.[17]

Health care workers involved in the direct patient care of patients who have had known, or suspected, exposure to the rabies virus should take standard precautions to ensure that they do not contract the virus from patients. Although no cases of transmission from patient to health care worker have been reported, proper prevention of exposure is warranted.[14] One report regarding a fatal human case of rabies estimated that standard precautions were not applied in 50% of health care workers having contact with the patient's bodily fluids, therefore necessitating the postexposure prophylaxis of multiple individuals.[81] Contact precautions, including barrier methods such as gloves, goggles, masks, and gowns, should be used to avoid contact with the patient's bodily substances, mucous membranes, or open wounds, which could theoretically lead to exposure.

MANAGEMENT AND REPORTING OF ADVERSE REACTIONS

With any medication therapy, adverse reactions do occur and the rabies vaccine and rabies immunoglobulin are no exception. Most of these reactions are local ones; however, they are common.[45–47] Injection site pain is the most common local reaction, occurring in up to 70% of patients.[48,49] Systemic hypersensitivity reactions and neurologic disorders are less frequent.[50–52] For local and mild adverse reactions, it is recommended that the rabies vaccination series should not be interrupted or discontinued. Attempts should be made to alleviate or mitigate these reactions through the use of additional pharmacotherapy modalities (ie, antiinflammatory, antihistaminic, and antipyretic agents).[17] Even in situations in which serious systemic hypersensitivity reactions occur, it is still necessary to carefully consider a patient's risk for acquiring rabies before discontinuing the vaccination series. It is recommended to seek the consultation of the CDC or state or local health officials to assist in the management of this challenging situation.[17]

In the unique situation of a patient with a previous history of hypersensitivity to the rabies vaccine who presents for revaccination, pretreatment with antihistamines, antiinflammatories, or H_2-antagonists should be considered. Because the risk of stimulating an anaphylactic reaction may be higher in this population, it is important to ensure that epinephrine is on hand during vaccination and careful monitoring is in place after vaccination.[82]

Adverse Event Reporting

It is imperative for the health care system to adequately document the occurrence of adverse events arising from the usage of medications and vaccines for multiple reasons, including quality control and safety, and to allow clinicians to have data to adequately weigh the risks and benefits of treating this often-indeterminate diagnosis. Clinically significant adverse events arising from the administration of the rabies vaccine should be reported to the Vaccine Adverse Event Reporting System

(VAERS).[83] The VAERS system is a CDC and FDA postmarketing surveillance tool for collecting adverse events secondary to US vaccines. VAERS submissions can be made online, by fax, or by email at http://www.vaers.hhs.gov or by telephone (800-822-7967). Adverse events after the use of HRIG administration should be reported to the FDA's MedWatch program. The MedWatch program was created for voluntary reporting of adverse events associated with drugs, biologics, medical devices, dietary supplements, or cosmetics. Reports of these reactions can be submitted online at http://www.fda.gov/Safety/MedWatch/HowToReport/default.htm.

SPECIAL POPULATIONS
Immunosuppression

It is possible that those patients who present with a history of a compromised immune system secondary to disease or pharmacotherapy (eg, systemic corticosteroids, immunosuppressive agents) may have an impaired ability to produce active immunity after vaccination.[84,85] Therefore, in cases of a finite term of immunosuppression such as systemic corticosteroids, it is recommended that preexposure prophylaxis be postponed and at-risk behavior be avoided, until the patient's immune system has recovered. However, if this strategy is not possible, or the immunosuppressed status is indefinite, preexposure prophylaxis may be administered and followed with an immediate assessment of the patient's virus neutralizing antibody titers. With regards to postexposure prophylaxis in this population, there have been no cases of therapy failure in this population. Postexposure prophylaxis should follow the ACIP recommendation of 5 total vaccine doses as opposed to the 4 recommended for otherwise healthy individuals. The administration of immunosuppressive agents should be avoided during the administration of the postexposure prophylaxis series unless deemed absolutely medically necessary. If this situation occurs, it is reasonable to assess rabies virus neutralizing antibody levels to ensure the development of active immunity.

Pregnancy

As a result of the high mortality risk of untreated rabies and the fact that studies have indicated no increased incidence of abortion, premature births, or fetal abnormalities associated with rabies vaccination, pregnancy is not considered a contraindication to postexposure prophylaxis.[86] However, both versions of the vaccine and HRIG are pregnancy category C. Preexposure prophylaxis may be indicated during pregnancy if the risk of rabies acquisition is high enough to warrant the ill-defined risk of vaccine administration.

COST

The direct and indirect medical costs associated with postexposure prophylaxis can be extensive. The CDC conducted a cost-effectiveness analysis to ascertain the costs of 8 contact scenarios. The cost of 1 dose of HRIG was estimated to be $326 to $1,434, 5 doses of vaccine $113 to $679 each, hospital charges $289 to $624, and physician charges $295 to $641.[17] Indirect costs such as travel, lost wages, alternative medicine, and other costs were estimated at $161 to $2161. The analysis determined that it always results in a cost savings to administer postexposure prophylaxis if a patient is bitten by a rabid animal that has tested positive for rabies or if a patient is bitten by a reservoir or vector species (eg, skunk, raccoon, bat, or fox bite in the United States or a dog bite in countries with dog variant rabies), even if the animal is not available for testing. For all other transmission risk situations, the average net cost-effectiveness ratio was always a net cost per life saved ranging from $2.9 million to $4 billion. This wide range reflects the lack of precise estimates regarding risk for transmission. The high cost of therapy underscores the necessity for a logical and systematic approach to accurately assessing the true risk of rabies infection with which each patient presents.

TREATMENT OF RABIES

In 2011, samples from 41 humans were submitted to the CDC for rabies evaluation, and 6 cases were confirmed.[21] This figure constitutes a total of 33 cases in the United States since 2002. Rabies is associated with the highest case fatality of any infectious disease, and survival has been documented in only a handful of patients.[17] Of those who have survived, almost all received some form of rabies vaccination before symptom onset.[87–92] Nevertheless, rabies is not considered a treatable disease, and treatment consists of nothing more than supportive care. After the onset of symptoms, patients die within days to weeks after presentation. To assist practitioners in the care of patients presenting with rabies, the Children's Hospital of Wisconsin has developed a rabies registry and provided a copy of their protocol for the treatment of patients with rabies (http://www.chw.org/display/ppf/docid/33223/router.asp).

Although there is no proven therapy for rabies, multiple medications have been used in futile attempts to stave off this disease, including the use of vidarabine, multisite vaccination with cell-culture vaccines, human leukocyte interferon, HRIG by the intravenous and intrathecal routes, antithymocyte globulin, inosine pranobex, ribavirin, ketamine, and high doses of steroids.[93–98] It has been determined that the administration of postexposure prophylaxis to a patient with clinical symptoms is ineffective and may be harmful.[70] In addition, HRIG should be avoided after the onset of symptoms, because it may interfere with the immune response to an active rabies infection that has already begun, and it cannot penetrate the blood-brain barrier and reach the site of infection.

Before initiating any investigational and aggressive therapy, a solid diagnosis of rabies should be confirmed with the CDC. In addition, the patient, provider, and family must recognize and understand that the likelihood of survival is low and that any survival will likely occur with serious neurologic sequelae. Those who have achieved better outcomes include those of a younger age, those with few or no concomitant medical conditions, vaccination before the onset of symptoms, and early presentation at the time of treatment initiation.[93] If the decision is made to treat, the treatment regimen involves a multipronged approach of supportive care, sedation, analgesics, anticonvulsants, and antivirals.[4,92,93,99]

Supportive care is the cornerstone of care for the patient infected with rabies, and standard critical care guidelines should be followed.[92] After stabilization of the patient, 1 approach that is often advocated is to induce a therapeutic coma in the patient.[92] The theory is that through this induced coma, cerebral ischemia secondary to hypermetabolic demands and seizure activity are reduced as well as decreasing any direct toxicity from sympathetic mediators. Some of the agents tested for this purpose include ketamine, benzodiazepines, barbiturates, and propofol.[72,92,100] Although all of these agents have provided some level of success with regards to inducing a therapeutic coma, with the overall limited survival associated with any therapy, there are no data to advocate for the use of 1 agent over another or for the therapeutic coma approach at all.

After stabilization of the patient and attempts to minimize the damage from the rabies virus, several antiviral agents have been used to target the virus itself. These agents include ribavirin, amantadine, interferon α, and acyclovir.[7,92] Because of the low success rates of all therapies, inadequate data are available to recommend 1 agent over another. However, available research does strongly support the concomitant use of 2 agents over monotherapy secondary to concerns over resistance or ineffectiveness.[93] The corollary is that with the use of multiple therapies comes an increased risk of adverse effects.[92,93] For example, ribavirin may cause hemolysis, mitochondrial toxicity, and pancreatitis, whereas interferon α may present its own neurotoxic effects. Despite multiple attempts with various agents, no antiviral agent can be recommended for the treatment of a human rabies infection.

SUMMARY

Rabies is a devastating encephalitis caused by a group of RNA viruses that use mammals as reservoirs. It is transmitted primarily through infected saliva contained in the bite of an infected mammal. In the United States, most naturally acquired human cases have come from bats. The use of appropriate preexposure and postexposure prophylaxis is critical and may be nearly 100% effective. If prophylaxis is not used, or is implemented incorrectly, then the patient may develop clinical rabies, which is almost universally fatal in humans. It is critical for all health care practitioners to be familiar with the appropriate evaluation of patients presenting with a possible rabies exposure and ensure that expeditious and appropriate prophylaxis is provided to help prevent the development of this lethal disease.

REFERENCES

1. Botvinkin AD, Poleschuk EM, Kuzmin IV, et al. Novel lyssaviruses isolated from bats in Russia. Emerg Infect Dis 2003;9:1623–5.
2. Fooks AR, Brookes SM, Johnson N, et al. European bat lyssaviruses: an emerging zoonosis. Epidemiol Infect 2003;131:1029–39.
3. World Health Organization. Rabies fact sheet. Geneva, Switzerland: World Health Organization; 2012.
4. Jackson AC. Recovery from rabies. N Engl J Med 2005;352:2549–50.
5. Anderson LJ, Nicholson KG, Tauxe RV, et al. Human rabies in the United States, 1960 to 1979: epidemiology, diagnosis, and prevention. Ann Intern Med 1984; 100:728–35.
6. Held JR, Tierkel ES, Steele JH. Rabies in man and animals in the United States, 1946-65. Public Health Rep 1967;82:1009–18.
7. Noah DL, Drenzek CL, Smith JS, et al. Epidemiology of human rabies in the United States, 1980 to 1996. Ann Intern Med 1998;128:922–30.
8. Warrell MJ, Warrell DA. Rabies and other lyssavirus diseases. Lancet 2004;363: 959–69.
9. Centers for Disease Control and Prevention. Rabies prevention. Atlanta, GA: Centers for Disease Control and Prevention; 2008.
10. Moran GJ, Talan DA, Mower W, et al. Appropriateness of rabies postexposure prophylaxis treatment for animal exposures. Emergency ID Net Study Group. JAMA 2000;284:1001–7.
11. Centers for Disease Control and Prevention. Cost of rabies prevention. Atlanta, GA: Centers for Disease Control and Prevention; 2008.
12. Hemachudha T, Laothamatas J, Rupprecht CE. Human rabies: a disease of complex neuropathogenetic mechanisms and diagnostic challenges. Lancet Neurol 2002;1:101–9.

13. King AA, Meredith CD, Thomson GR. The biology of southern African lyssavirus variants. Curr Top Microbiol Immunol 1994;187:267–95.
14. Rupprecht CE, Gibbons RV. Clinical practice. Prophylaxis against rabies. N Engl J Med 2004;351:2626–35.
15. Charlton KM. The pathogenesis of rabies and other lyssaviral infections: recent studies. Curr Top Microbiol Immunol 1994;187:95–119.
16. Leung AK, Davies HD, Hon KL. Rabies: epidemiology, pathogenesis, and prophylaxis. Adv Ther 2007;24:1340–7.
17. Manning SE, Rupprecht CE, Fishbein D, et al. Human rabies prevention–United States, 2008: recommendations of the Advisory Committee on Immunization Practices. MMWR Recomm Rep 2008;57:1–28.
18. Krebs JW, Mandel EJ, Swerdlow DL, et al. Rabies surveillance in the United States during 2004. J Am Vet Med Assoc 2005;227:1912–25.
19. Fekadu M. Canine rabies. Onderstepoort J Vet Res 1993;60:421–7.
20. Schneider MC, Belotto A, Ade MP, et al. Current status of human rabies transmitted by dogs in Latin America. Cad Saude Publica 2007;23:2049–63.
21. Blanton JD, Dyer J, McBrayer J, et al. Rabies surveillance in the United States during 2011. J Am Vet Med Assoc 2012;241:712–22.
22. Gibbons RV. Cryptogenic rabies, bats, and the question of aerosol transmission. Ann Emerg Med 2002;39:528–36.
23. Bronnert J, Wilde H, Tepsumethanon V, et al. Organ transplantations and rabies transmission. J Travel Med 2007;14:177–80.
24. Dietzschold B, Koprowski H. Rabies transmission from organ transplants in the USA. Lancet 2004;364:648–9.
25. Hellenbrand W, Meyer C, Rasch G, et al. Cases of rabies in Germany following organ transplantation. Euro Surveill 2005;10:E050224.6.
26. Messenger SL, Smith JS, Rupprecht CE. Emerging epidemiology of bat-associated cryptic cases of rabies in humans in the United States. Clin Infect Dis 2002;35:738–47.
27. Jackson AC. Rabies. Neurol Clin 2008;26:717–26, ix.
28. Srinivasan A, Burton EC, Kuehnert MJ, et al. Transmission of rabies virus from an organ donor to four transplant recipients. N Engl J Med 2005;352:1103–11.
29. Feder HM Jr, Petersen BW, Robertson KL, et al. Rabies: still a uniformly fatal disease? Historical occurrence, epidemiological trends, and paradigm shifts. Curr Infect Dis Rep 2012;14:408–22.
30. Rupprecht CE, Hanlon CA, Hemachudha T. Rabies re-examined. Lancet Infect Dis 2002;2:327–43.
31. Nigg AJ, Walker PL. Overview, prevention, and treatment of rabies. Pharmacotherapy 2009;29:1182–95.
32. Jackson AC, Ye H, Phelan CC, et al. Extraneural organ involvement in human rabies. Lab Invest 1999;79:945–51.
33. Meslin FX. Rabies as a traveler's risk, especially in high-endemicity areas. J Travel Med 2005;12(Suppl 1):S30–40.
34. Rupprecht CE, Briggs D, Brown CM, et al. Use of a reduced (4-dose) vaccine schedule for postexposure prophylaxis to prevent human rabies: recommendations of the advisory committee on immunization practices. MMWR Recomm Rep 2010;59:1–9.
35. Johnson N, Cunningham AF, Fooks AR. The immune response to rabies virus infection and vaccination. Vaccine 2010;28:3896–901.
36. Jackson AC. Rabies in the critical care unit: diagnostic and therapeutic approaches. Can J Neurol Sci 2011;38:689–95.

37. Warrell DA, Davidson NM, Pope HM, et al. Pathophysiologic studies in human rabies. Am J Med 1976;60:180–90.
38. Novartis. RabAvert rabies vaccine [package insert] Emeryville, CA: 2006.
39. Sanofi Pasteur. Imovax rabies vaccine [package insert] Swiftwater, PA: 2012.
40. Fishbein DB, Sawyer LA, Reid-Sanden FL, et al. Administration of human diploid-cell rabies vaccine in the gluteal area. N Engl J Med 1988;318:124–5.
41. Verma R, Khanna P, Prinja S, et al. Intra-dermal administration of rabies vaccines in developing countries: at an affordable cost. Hum Vaccin 2011;7:792–4.
42. WHO Expert Committee on Rabies. World Health Organ Tech Rep Ser 1992;824: 1–84.
43. Human rabies prevention–United States, 1999. Recommendations of the Advisory Committee on Immunization Practices (ACIP). MMWR Recomm Rep 1999;48:1–21.
44. Briggs DJ, Dreesen DW, Nicolay U, et al. Purified Chick Embryo Cell Culture Rabies Vaccine: interchangeability with Human Diploid Cell Culture Rabies Vaccine and comparison of one versus two-dose post-exposure booster regimen for previously immunized persons. Vaccine 2000;19:1055–60.
45. Ajjan N, Pilet C. Comparative study of the safety and protective value, in pre-exposure use, of rabies vaccine cultivated on human diploid cells (HDCV) and of the new vaccine grown on Vero cells. Vaccine 1989;7:125–8.
46. Arora A, Moeller L, Froeschle J. Safety and immunogenicity of a new chromatographically purified rabies vaccine in comparison to the human diploid cell vaccine. J Travel Med 2004;11:195–9.
47. Sabchareon A, Lang J, Attanath P, et al. A new Vero cell rabies vaccine: results of a comparative trial with human diploid cell rabies vaccine in children. Clin Infect Dis 1999;29:141–9.
48. Dreesen DW, Fishbein DB, Kemp DT, et al. Two-year comparative trial on the immunogenicity and adverse effects of purified chick embryo cell rabies vaccine for pre-exposure immunization. Vaccine 1989;7:397–400.
49. Deshpande AK, Londhe VA, Akarte S, et al. Comparative evaluation of immunogenicity, reactogenecity and safety of purified chick embryo cell rabies vaccine and neural tissue rabies vaccine. J Assoc Physicians India 2003;51:655–8.
50. Fishbein DB, Yenne KM, Dreesen DW, et al. Risk factors for systemic hypersensitivity reactions after booster vaccinations with human diploid cell rabies vaccine: a nationwide prospective study. Vaccine 1993;11:1390–4.
51. Bernard KW, Smith PW, Kader FJ, et al. Neuroparalytic illness and human diploid cell rabies vaccine. JAMA 1982;248:3136–8.
52. Boe E, Nyland H. Guillain-Barré syndrome after vaccination with human diploid cell rabies vaccine. Scand J Infect Dis 1980;12:231–2.
53. Cabasso VJ, Loofbourow JC, Roby RE, et al. Rabies immune globulin of human origin: preparation and dosage determination in non-exposed volunteer subjects. Bull World Health Organ 1971;45:303–15.
54. Talecris Biotherapeutics. HyperRAB S/D [package insert] Research Triangle Park, NC: 2010.
55. Sanofi Pasteur. Imogam rabies–HT [package insert] Swiftwater, PA: 2005.
56. Koprowski H, Van Der Scheer J, Black J. Use of hyperimmune anti-rabies serum concentrates in experimental rabies. Am J Med 1950;8:412–20.
57. Dean DJ, Baer GM, Thompson WR. Studies on the local treatment of rabies-infected wounds. Bull World Health Organ 1963;28:477–86.
58. Siber GR, Werner BG, Halsey NA, et al. Interference of immune globulin with measles and rubella immunization. J Pediatr 1993;122:204–11.

59. Atkinson WL, Pickering LK, Schwartz B, et al. General recommendations on immunization. Recommendations of the Advisory Committee on Immunization Practices (ACIP) and the American Academy of Family Physicians (AAFP). MMWR Recomm Rep 2002;51:1–35.
60. Lang J, Gravenstein S, Briggs D, et al. Evaluation of the safety and immunogenicity of a new, heat-treated human rabies immune globulin using a sham, post-exposure prophylaxis of rabies. Biologicals 1998;26:7–15.
61. LeGuerrier P, Pilon PA, Deshaies D, et al. Pre-exposure rabies prophylaxis for the international traveller: a decision analysis. Vaccine 1996;14:167–76.
62. Fishbein DB, Arcangeli S. Rabies prevention in primary care. A four-step approach. Postgrad Med 1987;82:83–90, 3–5.
63. Gautret P, Parola P. Rabies vaccination for international travelers. Vaccine 2012; 30:126–33.
64. Gautret P, Shaw M, Gazin P, et al. Rabies postexposure prophylaxis in returned injured travelers from France, Australia, and New Zealand: a retrospective study. J Travel Med 2008;15:25–30.
65. Hatz CF, Bidaux JM, Eichenberger K, et al. Circumstances and management of 72 animal bites among long-term residents in the tropics. Vaccine 1995;13:811–5.
66. Fishbein DB, Bernard KW, Miller KD, et al. The early kinetics of the neutralizing antibody response after booster immunizations with human diploid cell rabies vaccine. Am J Trop Med Hyg 1986;35:663–70.
67. Christian KA, Blanton JD, Auslander M, et al. Epidemiology of rabies post-exposure prophylaxis–United States of America, 2006-2008. Vaccine 2009;27: 7156–61.
68. Krebs JW, Long-Marin SC, Childs JE. Causes, costs, and estimates of rabies postexposure prophylaxis treatments in the United States. J Public Health Manag Pract 1998;4:56–62.
69. Dreesen DW, Bernard KW, Parker RA, et al. Immune complex-like disease in 23 persons following a booster dose of rabies human diploid cell vaccine. Vaccine 1986;4:45–9.
70. WHO Expert Consultation on rabies. World Health Organ Tech Rep Ser 2005; 931:1–88.
71. Kaplan MM, Cohen D, Koprowski H, et al. Studies on the local treatment of wounds for the prevention of rabies. Bull World Health Organ 1962;26:765–75.
72. McDermid RC, Saxinger L, Lee B, et al. Human rabies encephalitis following bat exposure: failure of therapeutic coma. CMAJ 2008;178:557–61.
73. Khawplod P, Wilde H, Chomchey P, et al. What is an acceptable delay in rabies immune globulin administration when vaccine alone had been given previously? Vaccine 1996;14:389–91.
74. Helmick CG, Johnstone C, Sumner J, et al. A clinical study of Merieux human rabies immune globulin. J Biol Stand 1982;10:357–67.
75. Wilde H, Sirikawin S, Sabcharoen A, et al. Failure of postexposure treatment of rabies in children. Clin Infect Dis 1996;22:228–32.
76. Rupprecht CE, Briggs D, Brown CM, et al. Evidence for a 4-dose vaccine schedule for human rabies post-exposure prophylaxis in previously non-vaccinated individuals. Vaccine 2009;27:7141–8.
77. Jenkins SR, Auslander M, Conti L, et al. Compendium of animal rabies prevention and control, 2004. J Am Vet Med Assoc 2004;224:216–22.
78. Thraenhart O, Marcus I, Kreuzfelder E. Current and future immunoprophylaxis against human rabies: reduction of treatment failures and errors. Curr Top Microbiol Immunol 1994;187:173–94.

79. Smith JS, Fishbein DB, Rupprecht CE, et al. Unexplained rabies in three immigrants in the United States. A virologic investigation. N Engl J Med 1991;324:205–11.
80. Helmick CG. The epidemiology of human rabies postexposure prophylaxis, 1980-1981. JAMA 1983;250:1990–6.
81. Mahamat A, Meynard JB, Djossou F, et al. Risk of rabies transmission and adverse effects of postexposure prophylaxis in health care workers exposed to a fatal case of human rabies. Am J Infect Control 2012;40:456–8.
82. Kroger AT, Atkinson WL, Marcuse EK, et al. General recommendations on immunization: recommendations of the Advisory Committee on Immunization Practices (ACIP). MMWR Recomm Rep 2006;55:1–48.
83. Varricchio F, Iskander J, Destefano F, et al. Understanding vaccine safety information from the vaccine adverse event reporting system. Pediatr Infect Dis J 2004;23:287–94.
84. Enright JB, Franti CE, Frye FL, et al. The effects of corticosteroids on rabies in mice. Can J Microbiol 1970;16:667–75.
85. Pappaioanou M, Fishbein DB, Dreesen DW, et al. Antibody response to preexposure human diploid-cell rabies vaccine given concurrently with chloroquine. N Engl J Med 1986;314:280–4.
86. Chutivongse S, Wilde H, Benjavongkulchai M, et al. Postexposure rabies vaccination during pregnancy: effect on 202 women and their infants. Clin Infect Dis 1995;20:818–20.
87. Recovery of a patient from clinical rabies–Wisconsin, 2004. MMWR Morb Mortal Wkly Rep 2004;53:1171–3.
88. Alvarez L, Fajardo R, Lopez E, et al. Partial recovery from rabies in a nine-year-old boy. Pediatr Infect Dis J 1994;13:1154–5.
89. Hattwick MA, Weis TT, Stechschulte CJ, et al. Recovery from rabies. A case report. Ann Intern Med 1972;76:931–42.
90. Madhusudana SN, Nagaraj D, Uday M, et al. Partial recovery from rabies in a six-year-old girl. Int J Infect Dis 2002;6:85–6.
91. Porras C, Barboza JJ, Fuenzalida E, et al. Recovery from rabies in man. Ann Intern Med 1976;85:44–8.
92. Willoughby RE Jr, Tieves KS, Hoffman GM, et al. Survival after treatment of rabies with induction of coma. N Engl J Med 2005;352:2508–14.
93. Jackson AC, Warrell MJ, Rupprecht CE, et al. Management of rabies in humans. Clin Infect Dis 2003;36:60–3.
94. Warrell MJ, White NJ, Looareesuwan S, et al. Failure of interferon alfa and tribavirin in rabies encephalitis. BMJ 1989;299:830–3.
95. Emmons RW, Leonard LL, DeGenaro F Jr, et al. A case of human rabies with prolonged survival. Intervirology 1973;1:60–72.
96. Hattwick MA, Corey L, Creech WB. Clinical use of human globulin immune to rabies virus. J Infect Dis 1976;133(Suppl):A266–72.
97. Kureishi A, Xu LZ, Wu H, et al. Rabies in China: recommendations for control. Bull World Health Organ 1992;70:443–50.
98. Merigan TC, Baer GM, Winkler WG, et al. Human leukocyte interferon administration to patients with symptomatic and suspected rabies. Ann Neurol 1984;16:82–7.
99. Hemachudha T, Sunsaneewitayakul B, Desudchit T, et al. Failure of therapeutic coma and ketamine for therapy of human rabies. J Neurovirol 2006;12:407–9.
100. Lockhart BP, Tordo N, Tsiang H. Inhibition of rabies virus transcription in rat cortical neurons with the dissociative anesthetic ketamine. Antimicrob Agents Chemother 1992;36:1750–5.

The Impact of Heat on Morbidity and Mortality

Stephen D. Krau, PhD, RN, CNE

KEYWORDS

- Heat morbidity • Heat mortality • Heat vulnerability • Heat early warning systems
- Heat-related risk factors • Exertional heat • Nonexertional heat

KEY POINTS

- Extreme heat poses risks for increases in heat-related morbidity, heat-related mortality, and expenditure of health care resources.
- Several risk factors associated with heat-related mortality include lack of air conditioning, single marital status, age, lower socioeconomic level, lower educational level, ethnicity, and preexisting medical conditions.
- Models for heat early warning systems are evident in several European countries.
- Living in urban areas poses higher risk for heat mortality than living in suburban or rural areas.
- Critical care nurses are uniquely poised to make an impact on the mortality and morbidity of persons at risk for heat-related health issues.

Summer weather is an invitation to engage in activities that are conducive to, and enhanced by, the warmer weather. Evidence exists that more people died as the result of heatstroke than the combined effects of hurricanes, lightning, earthquakes, floods, and tornadoes.[1] A culmination of factors contribute to the morbidity and mortality associated with heat conditions, including the heat index, the degree and type of exertion in which the individual engages, the overall health and wellness of the person in the warm summer sun, their location, and the resources available to these individuals. Heat-related mortality occurs in industrialized nations as well as those nations that are less developed.

During heat periods, there is an increased demand on health care services, including ambulance and hospital emergency services.[2] Such a demand has a definitive impact on the resources available to persons who endure heat-related emergencies, which could result in delays in response time, or even lack of available services where hospitals are on diversion. Epidemiologic literature related to heat-related issues has used a variety of methods to determine the impact of heat on morbidity and mortality. There are some variations across geographic and sociopolitical

School of Nursing, Vanderbilt University Medical Center, 461 21st Avenue South, Nashville, TN 37240, USA
E-mail address: steve.krau@vanderbilt.edu

Crit Care Nurs Clin N Am 25 (2013) 243–250
http://dx.doi.org/10.1016/j.ccell.2013.02.009
0899-5885/13/$ – see front matter © 2013 Elsevier Inc. All rights reserved.

boundaries, but for the most part, it is agreed that an increase in heat-related morbidities and mortalities is expected as a result of predicted temperature increases caused by worldwide climate change.[3–5]

WEATHER CONDITIONS

Most of the studies related to heat waves and weather conditions have been retrospective studies, in which data are collected after such events to determine the extent of heat-related illness that resulted in emergency room visits and mortalities. The association between high temperatures and mortality has been well documented, but the nonfatal causalities of heat have been less explored. In addition, there is some diversity in the measurement of the heat exposure that individuals endure. In addition to the ambient temperature, other factors such as sun exposure and its radiation effects, humidity, barometric pressure, and wind are considered part of the contributing features related to environmental heat measurement.[6–8]

A variety of measures that combine these effects have been used to develop occupational safety exposure guidelines and public health warning thresholds. Some of these measures include a heat index, a humidex, which is primary used in Canada, and wet bulb globe temperature (WBGT).[6] The WBGT is a sensor device that takes into account a variety of factors to determine the safe amount of time an individual can be outdoors on a hot day. The American Association of Pediatrics references the index from the WBGT readings to determine child safety measures on hot days. In addition, there are standards presented for athletes to stop training at certain indices, as well as indices for when military personnel should stop training.[9]

In attempts to capture the physiologic impact of the heat on an individual, some indices, such as the Physiologically Equivalent Temperature, have been considered.[3]

HEAT-ISLAND EFFECT

There is a phenomenon called heat-island effect, which describes the rationale behind urban areas having a higher temperature than their surrounding rural areas. In urban settings, the buildings and roads have replaced the open areas and the vegetation that once existed there. Because these structures are less permeable, and affect moisture, the area forms an island of higher temperatures. Heat islands occur on the surface of the atmosphere, where on hot, sunny summer days, urban surfaces such as roofs, roads, and pavements that are exposed to the sun can make temperatures 50° to 90°F hotter than the air.[10] Hence, the old adage, "It was so hot, you could fry eggs on the sidewalk"; one can! Typically, heat islands persist during the day and night, although they are most strong during the day, when the sun is shining. Heat islands contribute to persons in an urban setting being at a higher risk for heat-related vulnerability.[11]

Studies related to the heat-island effect have indicated that albedo, or reflectivity, of an urban setting is one of the most important determinants in the magnitude of the heat island.[12–14] Simulation studies related to city-wide albedo have shown that a reduction in albedo produces a modest, although significant, reduction in temperature.[14,15] The thought behind this model indicates that plants and vegetation on roofs and in areas throughout the urban setting would reduce the reflectivity and diminish the intensity and some of the effect of the heat island.

EXERTIONAL VERSUS NONEXERTIONAL HEAT-RELATED MORBIDITY

For further discussion, it is important to identify the context in which the person experiencing a heat-related issue is engaged. When a person who is essentially healthy is engaged in activities in the heat that bring about heat-related illnesses, caused by exertion or other factors that increase heat, the situation is referred to as exertional. When discussing heat stroke, the essentially healthy person is identified as having suffered exertional heat stroke. When an individual who has underlying medical issues or is on medications is exposed to heat without engaging in arduous activity and experiences a heat-related illness, this is referred to as nonexertional. Individuals who experience a heat stroke are identified as having classic heat stroke.

The distinction is important because the type of heat-related illness poses specific determinants. For example, exertional heat stroke is 1 of the top 3 leading causes of sudden death in athletes and is the leading cause of death of athletes during the months of July and August.[16] Increased ambient heat, along with decreased hydration, and heat retention resulting from uniforms and protective gear increase the likelihood of a heat-related issue. Also, the timing of the activity as it relates to the acclimatization of the athlete is a consideration. It is not unusual to see more issues during the first week of athletic activity than later in the practice trajectory.

EXERTIONAL HEAT ILLNESS

A national study indicated that most persons (66.1%) who suffered an exertional heat-related injury did so during the months of June, July, and August.[17]

Most exertional heat-related illness was associated with exercise and sporting activities (75.5%), followed by yard work (11.0%), home maintenance activities (4.6%), and other recreational activities such as swimming and playing on the playground (3.8%).[17] During this study from 1997 to 2006, about 48% of those identified as having exertional heat-related illness had exact diagnoses. In those for whom information was available, 72.7% were diagnosed with heat exhaustion, and 18.7% were diagnosed with dehydration, followed by heat syncope (9.7%), heat cramps (5.4%), heat stress (1.9%), and heat stroke (1.8%).[17]

Nearly half of the exertional heat illnesses occurred in children and adolescents. This finding is not surprising considering that these age groups do not adapt to extremes in temperatures as well as adults. Several physiologic characteristics contribute to this situation, along with the predisposition not to feel thirsty and replenish fluids, because hydration is an important determinant in heat illness.[17]

Next to football activities, golf accounted for 1 of the top 5 activities that induced heat-related illness for both men and women aged 20 years to older than 65 years.[17] Golf requires exposure to weather and the sun for long periods, and most courses are limited in shade to avoid obstructing the process of the game. Because this sport is popular with elderly adults, who are more vulnerable to heat-related issues, golf accounts for an increasing proportion of heat-related illness with age.[17]

Another factor that poses an issue for elderly people was reported in a recent study by Sheridan[18] related to heat warnings and advisories. The study was a multicity study that indicated that persons aged 65 years and older are unaware of protective actions to take during heat events. The respondents did acknowledge the existence of heat warnings, but did not consider themselves vulnerable to the heat. They did not consider that hot weather was a threat to their health, and only 46% modified their behavior on heat advisory days.[18] There are many implications for education and community services in these findings.

MORTALITY DISPLACEMENT

Mortality displacement, or harvesting, embodies the notion that deaths related to extremes in temperature are already expected among certain individuals who are frailer to advance mortality. As a result, these individuals are not considered to have significantly shortened lives as a result of heat or cold conditions.[3] This is an important concept when determining the mortality associated with extreme heat and contributes to an overall increase in numbers of deaths. This issue also comes into play when discussing deaths associated with pollution levels.[19] This issue is important when interpreting research results related to weather and pollution conditions. Variations in subgroups of populations in cities and geographic areas make the demographics of the study group and area important. This phenomenon is not a rationale for minimizing prevention or treatment to certain individuals. Mortality displacement is a hypothetical concept that confounds research and research findings. There are no practice implications or judgments for this phenomenon, other than in the interpretation of data analysis.

IDENTIFYING VULNERABLE POPULATIONS

Numerous retrospective studies examine variant demographic variables as they relate to heat-related illness and heat-related mortality.[11,20–26] Factors related to exertional heat-related injuries have been discussed. **Table 1** is an overview of some of the variations that affect morbidity and mortality outcomes related to heat.

RESOURCES AND ACTIONS

Using the factors that contribute to mortality and morbidity associated with heat, agencies can map areas of high vulnerability for heat-related issues.[32] Heat vulnerability varies spatially on a local, national, and international level. Mapping such effects is the first step in the planning of adaptive change as the climate changes. It is important for the critical care nurse to identify the factors in their community, because what occurs in any intensive care unit is often a reflection of what is occurring outside the walls of the hospital in the community.

In Europe, as a result of catastrophic heat events in the last few decades, there has been a concerted effort to develop heat wave early warning systems (HEWSs).[33] These systems involve early forecasting of heat waves, predicting potential health outcomes, prompting timely and effective response plans, as well as evaluating and communication about the system. The HEWS is similar to disaster planning in the United States, but targeted for those issues involving heat. These systems are designed to reduce potential human health consequences. They engage in a great deal of education related to heat wave and personal implications that heat waves may have on the individual. There is already clear evidence that there is a knowledge deficit among elderly people in the United States related to the personal impact that heat may have on them.[18]

Cities like Philadelphia and Phoenix have developed programs to act preventively and proactively in adapting to the impact that heat might have on the health of their citizens. However, initiatives such as these programs are not widespread. Such initiatives would provide useful plans for allocation of resources, including access to intensive care units.

Actions that warrant consideration by the critical care nurse first include enhancement of the personal knowledge of heat and heat-related illness. It is important to identify which conditions pose the most risk for heat-related illnesses, and which medications predispose the patient to heat-related illnesses. Then the nurse during the summer months can educate and support the patient in their health management during times of extreme heat. When considering the patient's living conditions, offering suggestions for temporary accommodation in the area and support for a cool environment would be helpful for those at risk.

Table 1
Factors that affect heat-related injuries

Factor	Relevance
Age	Children: small body mass/surface ratio along with greater susceptibility to dehydration makes them vulnerable to heat-related mortality and morbidity[5,25] Older adults: individuals 65 years and older are more sensitive to temperature extremes, particularly heat.[21,25] Elderly individuals are more likely to have medical conditions that increase risk for heat-related illnesses and mortality
Preexisting medical conditions	A variety of conditions and medications are associated with certain conditions that put certain individuals at a higher risk.[26] Many medications increase the risk of heat-related illness. Persons with cancer, cardiovascular conditions, limited mobility, diabetes,[3] and mental illnesses are at high risk. Persons on diuretics or medications that cause diuresis are more susceptible to dehydration
Geographic location	Living in areas where extreme heat is rare increases the risk of heat-related mortality.[27] This risk could be the result of lack of acclimatization or lack of available resources for extreme heat
Urban/rural	Higher vulnerability exists in metropolitan areas as opposed to their surrounding rural areas.[14] Higher vulnerability, regardless of air conditioning, existed in the downtown cores of cities[11]
Living in a nursing or care home	In the United Kingdom, it has been shown that persons living in nursing homes or skilled care facilities are more vulnerable to heat-related mortality[28]
Air conditioning	Areas with higher air conditioning prevalence have lower or no heat-related mortality.[14,29,30] During the 1995 Chicago heat waves, the incidence of dying was 70% less among persons with working air conditioners than persons without working air conditioners.[22] (An important issue here is the possibility of a power outage)
Socioeconomic status	Persons at or near the national poverty level are at increased risk for heat-related deaths[11]
Level of education	Persons with at most a high school education are at a higher risk of heat-related mortality than persons with more education[21]
Marital status	People who are married are less likely to die from heat compared with those who are widowed, divorced, or single.[11] A study after the heat wave in Chicago reported that people who lived alone, or did not leave home each day, had a higher risk of death than those with social contacts and access to transportation[22]
Race or ethnicity	In several studies, it has been shown that African Americans or blacks are at higher risk for heat-related morbidity and mortality, than whites.[11] In a recent study, blacks had a higher mortality than whites, but both had higher rates than Hispanics
Heat duration	Mortality has been found to increase during periods of 3 or more days of unusually hot temperatures in summer[31]
Occupational groups	Although this category may cross the nomenclature boundary into exertional heat-related incidents, by virtue of spending time outdoors during extreme heat, certain occupations are at risk. Outdoor workers in rural and suburban areas are at risk[25]

Outside the hospital in professional organizations and functions, it would be helpful for the critical care nurse to discuss heat issues with colleagues and other health care professionals to share ideas and experiences. Discussions would include appropriate first-aid response and use of heat safety action plans. Some of the community resources that might be considered are social workers, emergency shelters, police, and faith organizations.

During heat waves, it is important to not only monitor patient status to prevent rapid deterioration but also to keep vigilant of the family members who may be exposed to unusually high ambient heat. With the stresses that can accompany having a family member in a critical care area, family members are already predisposed to fatigue, alterations in eating, and hydration. This situation, accompanied by high ambient heat, puts the family member at risk for heat-related illness.

SUMMARY

Heat waves greatly increase the risk of death and serious illness among all sectors of society. Those with poor physical health, who work or play outdoors, or take certain medications are at particular risk. Heat vulnerability varies from patient to patient, and risk factors should be identified, particularly for patients who return home during times of inordinate heat. Risks are exacerbated because of a variety of socioeconomic, and individual factors. The factors warrant the consideration of the critical care nurse, not just for the patients for whom they care but also for the family members of those patients.

Critical care nurses have an obligation to increase the capabilities and hardiness of their patients to manage their illnesses during inordinate hot weather. Social services and organizations need to be aware of clients at risk to afford them immediate interventions when their patients lack the capacity or resources to maintain optimal levels of well-being during times of extreme heat and heat waves.

REFERENCES

1. Centers for Disease Control and Prevention (CDC). Heat-related mortality Arizona 1993-2002. And United States, 1979-2002. MMWR Morb Mortal Wkly Rep 2005; 54:628–30.
2. Nitschke M, Tucker GR, Bi P. Morbidity and mortality during heatwaves in metropolitan Adelaide. Med J Aust 2007;187(11–12):662–5.
3. O'Neill MS, Ebi KL. Temperature extremes and health: impacts of climate variability and change in the United States. J Occup Environ Med 2009;51(1):13–25.
4. Frumkin H, Hess J, Luber G, et al. Climate change: the public health response. Am J Public Health 2008;98(3):435–45.
5. Kovats RS, Hajat S. Heat stress and public health: a critical review. Annu Rev Public Health 2008;29:41–5.
6. Perry AG, Korenberg MJ, Hall GG, et al. Modeling and syndromic surveillance for estimating weather induced heat-related illness. J Environ Public Health 2011; 2011:1–10.
7. Steadman RG. The assessment of sultriness-part II: effects of wind, extra radiation and barometric pressure on apparent temperature. J Appl Meteorol 1979; 18(7):874–85.
8. Smoyer-Tomic KE, Rainham DG. Beating the heat: development and evaluation of Canadian hot weather health-response plan. Environ Health Perspect 2001; 109(12):1241–8.

9. Dimiceli VE, Piltz SF, Amburn SA. Estimation of Black Globe Temperature for calculation of the Wet Bulb Globe Temperature Index. Proceedings of the World Congress on Engineering and Computer Science 2011 vol. II, WCECS 2011. San Francisco, October 19–21, 2011.

10. Berdahl P, Bretz S. Preliminary survey of the solar reflectance of cool roofing materials. Energ Build 1997;25:149–58.

11. Reid CE, O'Neill MS, Gronlund CJ, et al. Mapping community determinants of heat vulnerability. Environ Health Perspect 2009;117(11):1730–6.

12. Kolokotroni M, Giridharan R. Urban heat island intensity in London: an investigation of the impact of physical characteristics on changes in the outdoor air temperature during summer. Sol Energ 2008;82(11):986–98.

13. Lynn BH, Carlso TN, Rosenzwieg C, et al. A modification to the NOAHLSM to simulate heat migration strategies in the New York City Metropolitan Area. J Appl Meteorol Climatol 2009;48(2):199–216.

14. O'Neill MS, Carter R, Kish JK, et al. Preventing heat-related morbidity and mortality: new approaches in a changing climate. Maturitas 2009;64(2):98–103.

15. Taha H. Meso-urban meteorological and photochemical modeling of heat island mitigation. Atmos Environ 2008;42(38):8795–809.

16. Pagnotta KD, Maderolle SM, Casa DJ. Exertional heat stroke and emergency issues in high school sport. J Strength Cond Res 2010;24(7):1707–9.

17. Nelson NG, Collins CL, Comstock RD, et al. Exertional heat-related injuries treated in emergency departments in the U.S., 1997-2006. Am J Prev Med 2011;40(1):54–60.

18. Sheridan SC. A survey of public perception and response to heat warnings across four North American cities: an evaluation of municipal effectiveness. Int J Biometeorol 2007;52:3–15.

19. Thomas D. Why do estimates of the acute and chronic effects of air pollution on mortality differ? J Toxicol Environ Health A 2005;68:1167–74.

20. Michelozzi P, Accetta G, DeSario M, et al. High temperature and hospitalizations for cardiovascular and respiratory causes in 12 European cities. Am J Respir Crit Care Med 2009;179(5):383–9.

21. Medina-Ramon M, Zanobetti A, Cavanagh DP, et al. Extreme temperatures and mortality: assessing effect modification of personal characteristics and specific cause of death in a multi-city case-only analysis. Environ Health Perspect 2006;114(9):1331–6.

22. Semenza JC, Rubin CH, Falter KH, et al. Heat-related deaths during the July 1995 heat wave in Chicago. N Engl J Med 1996;335:84–90.

23. O'Neill MS, Zanobetti A, Schwartz J. Disparities by race in heat-related mortality in four U.S. cities: the role of air conditioning prevalence. J Urban Health 2005;82: 191–7.

24. Sister C, Golden J, Chuang WC, et al. Mapping social vulnerability to heat wave in Chicago. In: The 89th American Meterological Society Annual Meeting. Phoenix, 2009 January 10–15.

25. Balbus JM. Identifying vulnerable subpopulations for climate change health effects in the United States. J Occup Environ Med 2009;51(1):33–7.

26. Hausfater P, Megarbane B, Dautheville S, et al. Prognostic factors in non-exertional heatstroke. Intensive Care Med 2010;36:272–80.

27. Kalkstein LS. Saving lives during extreme weather in summer. BMJ 2000;321: 650–1.

28. Hajat S, Kovats R, Lachowycz K. Heat-related and cold-related deaths in England and Wales: who is at risk? Environ Med 2007;64:93–100.

29. Anderson GB, Bell ML. Weather-related mortality: a study of how heat, cold and heat waves affect mortality in the United States. Epidemiology 2009;20(2): 205–13.

30. Basu R, Ostro BD. A multicountry analysis identifying the populations vulnerable to mortality associated with high ambient temperature in California. Am J Epidemiol 2008;168(6):632–7.

31. O'Neill MS, Zanobetti A, Schwartz J. Modifiers of the temperature and mortality association in seven U.S. cities. Am J Epidemiol 2003;157:1074–82.

32. Reid CE, Mann JK, Alfasso R, et al. Evaluation of a heat vulnerability index on abnormally hot days: an environmental public health tracking study. Environ Health Perspect 2012;120(5):715–20.

33. Lowe D, Ebi KL, Forsberg B. Heatwave early warning systems and adaptation advice to reduce human health consequences of heatwaves. Int J Environ Res Public Health 2011;8:4623–48.

Heat-Related Illness
A Hot Topic in Critical Care

Stephen D. Krau, PhD, RN, CNE

KEYWORDS

- Hyperthermia • Heatstroke • Heat exhaustion • Heat illness
- Multiple organ dysfunction • Disseminated intravascular coagulopathy
- Systemic inflammation response

KEY POINTS

- With current predictions of climate change, the incidence of heat-related illnesses is projected to increase.
- Heat-related illnesses occur on a continuum from mild symptoms to fatalities.
- To prevent heat-related illnesses, nurses should have comprehension of persons at risk.
- Primary treatment of heat-related illness centers on cooling, but not overcooling, the patient.
- Heatstroke involves coagulopathies and cytokines, and can result in systemic inflammatory response syndrome and multiple organ dysfunction.
- Critical care nursing intervention requires more than effective cooling to support bodily processes that have been damaged or destroyed by the pathophysiology of heatstroke.

Under current predictions of climate change, ambient heat conditions such as heat waves and hot weather are predicted to increase in frequency. Temperature extremes and variability are important determinants of health in the United States.[1] Every critical care nurse knows that what occurs within the intensive care areas is a reflection of happenings that occur outside the walls of the hospital. Exposure to hot weather, particularly during the summer months, is considered one of the most deadly natural hazards in the United States, particularly in unacclimatized and immunocompromised individuals.[2] Summer weather is an invitation to engage in activities that are conducive to, and enhanced by, the warmer weather. It was estimated that between 1979 and 2002 more people died as the result of heatstroke than the combined effects of hurricanes, lightning, earthquakes, floods, and tornadoes.[3] Because of the intricacies associated with heat-related illnesses, it is often processes that follow heatstroke itself

Disclosures: None.
School of Nursing, Vanderbilt University Medical Center, 461 21st Avenue South, 309 Godchaux Hall, Nashville, TN 37240, USA
E-mail address: steve.krau@vanderbilt.edu

Crit Care Nurs Clin N Am 25 (2013) 251–262
http://dx.doi.org/10.1016/j.ccell.2013.02.012
0899-5885/13/$ – see front matter © 2013 Elsevier Inc. All rights reserved.

that result in patient mortality. Risk factors, pathophysiologic pathways initiated by heat illnesses, and persons at risk are salient factors that warrant the understanding of critical care nurses who care for these patients.

HEAT-RELATED ILLNESS CONTINUUM

Heat-related illnesses constitute a continuum of pathologic conditions and have an impact on very diverse populations and persons of all demographics. When the heat index is exceeds 35°C (95°F), mortality increases proportionally not only to the elevation but also the duration of the elevation.[4,5] There is a variety of types of heat-related injuries including heat cramps, heat syncope, heat exhaustion, heat stress, and heatstroke.[6] Outcomes of these injuries can range from minor discomfort to mortality.

Illnesses associated with heat are best considered along a continuum of transition from heat intolerance, to a fairly mild condition of heat intolerance, to heat exhaustion, to heatstroke.[7] Milder forms of heat-related illnesses are typically associated with a core temperature of less than 40°C (104°F) with no apparent central nervous system symptoms.[8,9] An overview of the heat illness continuum with physiologic foundations, patient symptoms, and management strategies is presented in **Table 1**.

CLASSIFICATIONS OF HEATSTROKE: CLASSIC AND EXERTIONAL

When discussing heatstroke, it is important to identify the proper classification of the phenomenon. Although the physiologic bases of both are similar, the classification refers to the preexisting factors that contribute to the heatstroke. Classic heatstroke is primarily observed in persons with preexisting medical conditions or persons on certain medications who, when exposed to hot weather, experience heatstroke. Exertional heatstroke (EHS) occurs primarily in otherwise healthy individuals who are engaged in physical exertion during warm weather. Untreated EHS has a greater likelihood of morbidity and mortality because it is more prone to the development of rhabdomyolysis, renal failure, liver failure, electrolyte imbalances, and hypoglycemia.[10] There are certain medications that predispose an individual to classic heatstroke, listed in **Table 2**.

PHYSIOLOGIC BASIS

Body heat is the function of not only ambient or environmental heat but also the result of metabolic processes that occur in the human body. Thermoregulation of the body, however, assures that the body's core temperature is maintained at around 37°C (98.6°F). To this end, the receptors in the skin and viscera communicate with the temperature-sensitive neurons in the anterior and ventromedial hypothalamus and preoptic areas, as well as the mid-brain, brainstem, and spinal cord.[11,12] Thermoregulation is a dynamic process whereby increased body temperature results in an increased activation of these neurons, whereas a decrease in body temperature results in a decrease in neuron activation.

When an individual is hyperthermic, the body responds by increasing blood flow via vasodilation to the viscera and the periphery, thereby allowing heat loss through the process referred to as convection.[11] Skin is the major heat-dissipating organ, and increased blood flow increases heat loss.[13] Sweating and moving to a cooler area facilitate heat loss by the process known as evaporation. The amount of heat loss that occurs through sweating is influenced by both ambient temperature and atmospheric humidity. Hence, the geographic location of the individual, and the season,

Table 1
The heat illness continuum: from mild to severe signs and symptoms

Heat Illness	Physiologic Basis	Patient Symptoms	Management
Heat intolerance	Sense of feeling hot, and can cause sweating. Gradual onset; long duration	Inability to be comfortable with rising ambient heat	Air-conditioning (works better than fans) and hydration
Heat edema	Transient peripheral vasodilation from the heat	Swelling of the extremities, often accompanied by facial flushing. Clothing may feel restrictive, sweating and feeling of feeling hot and uncomfortable	Move to cooler place, hydrate, and elevate edematous extremity to reduce swelling
Heat rash	Typically the result of excessive sweating during heated conditions when the sweat ducts become blocked	Red cluster of pimples or small blisters. More likely to occur on neck, upper chest, groin, under the breasts, and in elbow creases	Remove clothing around area. Let the area air-dry instead of using towels. Avoid the use over-the-counter ointment and solutions, as this can irritate skin. If it persists, seek primary care provider's advice
Heat cramps	Usually result of fluid and electrolyte depletion. Can occur in any setting but most usually in hot and humid environments	Muscle spasms (usually abdomen, legs, or arms), moist and cool skin, normal or slightly elevated pulse, and normal body temperature	Rest, prolonged stretching of affected muscle group, and oral ingestion of fluids containing sodium. Intravenous normal saline sometimes used for rapid relief when patient cannot swallow
Heat syncope Heat syncope is an actual diagnosis	Lack of perfusion to the brain due to excessive exercise (decreased central venous blood return or dehydration)	Light-headedness, orthostasis, dizziness, fainting. Typically following exertion, and/or lack of acclimatization to the warm environment	Protect airway, move to cooler environment. Hydrate with clear liquids such as fruit juice, sports drinks, or diluted tea. Tepid bath
Heat exhaustion Heat exhaustion, unlike heat syncope, is a syndrome	Warning that the body is getting too hot and is typically the result of the body's loss of water and sodium	Thirst, headache, gooseflesh, giddiness, weakness, loss of coordination, nausea, diarrhea, profuse sweating, cold and clammy skin. Skin may be pale or ashen with associated hypotension	Remove excess clothing, and move to cool or shaded environment. Supine position, preferably with legs elevated. Oral fluids are preferable for those who can swallow and not nauseated or vomiting
Heatstroke	Multiform physiologic basis. Activation of cytokines and coagulopathies	Defined by elevated temperature and central nervous systems. Must contain both elements	Cooling is the gold standard of treatment. Support of affected organs and processes in prolonged or extreme cases

Table 2
Medications and substances that contribute to heat-related illness

Ecstasy	Morphine	Alcohol	Diuretics	Phenothiazines
Neuroleptics	Cocaine	Phenothiazides	Methamphetamines	Angiotensin-converting enzyme inhibitors
α-Adrenergic agonists	Ephedra-containing medications	Anticholinergics	Thyroid receptor agonists	Serotonin and noradrenaline reuptake inhibitors
Antihistamines	Benzodiazepines	β-Blockers	Calcium-channel blockers	Serotonin-specific uptake inhibitors
Amphetamines	Tricyclic antidepressants (older)	Caffeine	Laxatives	Desflurane
Neuroleptics	Methyldopa	Halothane	Sevoflurane	Succinylcholine

play an important role in thermoregulation. The mechanisms by which the body regulates heat are presented in **Table 3**.

THERMAL REGULATION: THE COMPENSATORY PHASE

Thermal regulation in heat situations occurs when the periphery vasodilates to enhance conductive heat loss into the atmosphere. As this process continues to

Table 3
Mechanisms of heat gain and loss

Mechanism	Description of Process	Considerations
Conduction	Transfer of heat between 2 surfaces with different temperatures that are in direct contact, eg, the exchange between a person's skin and clothing	The degree of conduction depends on the temperature gradient, the conductive properties of the object in contacting the body, and the percentage of the body that is in contact with the object
Convection	Transfer of heat between the surface of the body and a gas or fluid with a differing temperature, eg, a person being in a temperature that is freezing, or in ambient temperature that is much higher than body temperature	Convective heat exchange increases with increasing air speed and larger gradient between the air and skin temperature. Clothing that is permeable to air or that is loose fitting also increases convective heat loss
Radiation	Transfer of heat in the form of electromagnetic waves between the body and its surroundings, eg, a body that is being warmed by direct sunlight	Radiant energy is typically either reabsorbed or reflected, which is why light-colored clothing can help prevent heat-related illness. Light-colored clothing absorbs less heat
Evaporation	Conversion of a liquid, such as sweat, to a gaseous state such as water vapor	Depends on the integrity of skin, sweat production, and water-pressure gradient. As ambient humidity increases, this mechanism becomes less effective

maintain central perfusion, a peripheral vasoconstriction also occurs, thus allowing the body sufficient volume to maintain adequate blood pressure. One must keep in mind that if the individual is dehydrated or sweating profusely, there is already a chance of hypovolemia. In addition, there are adjustments in cardiovascular activity whereby the cardiovascular system transfers heat from the core and muscles to the body surface.[14] Sympathetic mediated cutaneous vasodilation concomitant with splanchnic vasoconstriction can increase cardiac output to 20 to 25 L/m.[14,15] The shunting of blood from the central circulation to the periphery reduces the perfusion to the viscera, particularly the kidney and intestines. The lack of perfusion to the kidney results in conservation of the body's fluids, as fluid loss occurs primarily through the skin and, to some extent, the respiratory system. In addition, the lack of perfusion to the intestines provides the physiologic bases for the occurrence of abdominal cramping, nausea, and/or vomiting, some of the earlier signs on the heat illness continuum.

THERMAL REGULATION: ACUTE-PHASE RESPONSE

When a person's core body temperature reaches or exceeds 40°C (104°F), cellular damage occurs. This process results in a coordinated reaction involving endothelial cells, leukocytes, and epithelial cells, which protects against further injury and promotes cellular repair.[14,16] In addition, release of protective proteins or heat shock proteins regulates the tissue reaction from potentially lethal stresses including "heat, ischemia, hypoxia, endotoxin, physical activity, oxidative stress, and others."[14] These proteins work in a variety of ways but primarily exert their protective effect by reinforcing the integrity of the epithelial barrier, thus preventing endotoxin leakage in the intestine by enhancing arterial blood pressure to reduce cerebral ischemia and neural damage, by ameliorating oxidative stress and obstructing the apoptotic cell-signaling pathways, and by affecting other proteins.[14]

THERMOREGULATORY FAILURE (THE UNCOMPENSATED PHASE)

This phase leads to the occurrence of heatstroke, which can lead to multiorgan dysfunction syndrome. These results constitute the focus for the critical care nurse. Whereas milder and more innocuous forms of heat illness are important for the critical care nurse to consider, it is persons with heatstroke that the nurse in a critical unit will more frequently encounter. The phase is associated with an intricate and dynamic interaction of acute physiologic processes associated with hyperthermia, which include circulatory failure, hypoxia, and increases in metabolic demand. In addition, direct cell suppression and cytotoxicity of heat, failure of the coagulation system, and systemic inflammatory response follow.[7,14,17,18]

Heat stress results in sweating, which is commensurate to fluid loss. The loss of fluid, if not replenished, can result in hypovolemia and a reduction cardiac output, as the compensatory system is no longer effective. The reduction of blood volume caused by dehydration, coupled with the diversion of blood to periphery and cutaneous areas, further reduces central venous pressure. Dehydration is not typically the direct cause of heatstroke; however, it may attenuate heat transfer and lead to cardiovascular collapse.[14] Sweating is a potential determinant in whether the patient has experienced a classic heatstroke or an exertional heatstroke. Patients with classic heatstroke are those who become more dehydrated because of medications or an underlying illness that impairs thermoregulation. Exertional heatstroke results from activity of an essentially healthy person in a warm environment. The cessation of sweating is a more common occurrence in classic heatstroke than in exertional heatstroke.[19]

During this phase the central venous pressure decreases. With this decrease, the ability to transfer body heat to the body surface is decreased, which results in an increase in core body temperature. This circulatory compromise contributes to thermoregulatory failure and to the advent of heatstroke. This process is accompanied by further blood shifts from the mesenteric circulation to the skin and working muscles, promoting ischemia and hyperpermeability of the intestines.[14] In addition, there is a concurrent increase in anaerobic metabolism, impaired clearance of lactic acid, and an overall systemic acidosis.[14] The damaged cell membranes allow the leakage of endotoxins into the vascular spaces, producing a shock syndrome characterized by hypotension, tachycardia, and inadequate organ perfusion.[20,21] When heat-stress conditions are severe, the reduction in hepatic portal circulation, combined with hepatocytes that are compromised by the heat itself, drastically reduces the ability of the liver to detoxify the growing surge of endotoxins.[22] The body becomes overwhelmed by the endotoxins.

This process accelerates the production and release of more cytokines, which provokes activation of endothelial cells and the release of vasoactive factors such as nitric oxide and endothelins.[14] These factors combine and create a potentially fatal cycle that is evidenced in heatstroke by very high body temperature and circulatory failure. In addition, the increase in cytokines is associated with high intracranial pressures, diminished cerebral blood flow, and severe injury to the neurons.[14,20] The ability to thermoregulate is further compromised by damage to the brain-center functions caused by the cerebral edema, blood-brain barrier dysfunction, and the release of endogenous pyrogens. The downward spiral the patient is experiencing is very apparent but continuous.

There follows a deterioration of cellular energy that induces a metabolic cascade, resulting in permanent cell damage.[23,24] This damage leads to cellular energy depletion, which contributes to worsening pathophysiology of heatstroke. Epstein and Roberts[14] explain this process in relation to a buildup of lactic acids as a result of cellular energy requirements, identifying that this increased requirement stimulates the adenosine triphosphate (ATP)-dependent sodium and potassium pump. The activity of the pump results in the production of more heat and, in the presence of compromised mitochondrial respiratory function, further reduces cellular energy levels. The depletion of ATP contributing to the compromise of the ion-transport systems leads to calcium accumulation which, in combination with lactic acid accumulation, contributes to further cell hypoxia and necrosis.[14,25,26]

In addition, a variety of mechanisms is mediated by thermoregulation, including potassium balance. During hyperthermia there is an increase in extracellular and intravascular potassium, as there is a tremendous loss of potassium within the cells.[27,28] Severe hyperthermia also results in an increase in intracellular calcium via a variety of transport mechanisms.[27,28]

HEATSTROKE AND COAGULOPATHIES

Disseminated intravascular coagulation (DIC) is a common complication associated with 45% of patients who experience heatstroke.[11] DIC in heatstroke is the result of thermal injury to the endothelium, and is an important contributor to the morbidity and mortality associated with heatstroke. Studies have shown that heat (43°–44°C [109.5°–111°F]) activates platelet aggregation, resulting in irreversible hyperaggregation following cooling.[29,30] Early in the process of a heatstroke there is an excess deposition of fibrin, particularly in the arterioles, which is the result of the widespread activation of coagulation stimulated by the heatstroke. Rapid cooling may normalize fibrinolysis, but the coagulation may persist until the patient's platelets and coagulation proteins are used faster than they are produced.[7,31] This form of coagulopathy can lead to excessive bleeding and is associated with high mortality rates. Endotoxins and cytokines are thought to amplify and participate in the progression of DIC by their effect on the leukocytes and endothelial cells.[7]

HEATSTROKE AND ACID-BASE IMBALANCE

Patients with heatstroke present with a variety and mixed acid-base disturbances. Predominant disturbances identified on admission are metabolic acidosis as the most prominent, followed by respiratory alkalosis.[11,32] The prevalence of metabolic acidosis, and not respiratory alkalosis, is contingent on the degree of hyperthermia (42°–43°C [107.5°–109.5°F]). Simple respiratory alkalosis is associated with persons who experience a lesser degree of hyperthermia. Although the actual mechanism for respiratory alkalosis is not clear, it is thought to be the result of an increase in alveolar ventilation independent of hypotension, hypoxemia, or other processes.[32] The metabolic acidosis is the result of the accumulation of lactic acid resulting from metabolic processes that occur throughout the body during heatstroke.

HEATSTROKE AND MULTIORGAN FAILURE

Two clinical findings must be present for the patient to be diagnosed with heatstroke, the first of which is hyperthermia, whereby the core body temperature may range from 40° to 47°C (104°–116.5°F).[20] The other mandatory presentation must include signs of central nervous system dysfunction. The brain dysfunction may be severe or subtle.[20] Symptoms of cerebral involvement might include confusion, overall mental status changes, delirium, combativeness, seizures, and coma. A variety of serious complications is associated with heatstroke, for which the critical care nurse must monitor. **Table 4** identifies the potential complications associated with heatstroke. It is important for the critical care nurse to realize that even though hyperthermia is the catalyst for the pathway leading to heatstroke, the fatal outcome of heatstroke is related to the ensuing multiorgan failure and complications that occur, as presented in **Table 4**.

TREATMENT AND MANAGEMENT OF HEATSTROKE

Heatstroke is more preventable than treatable. Identification of persons at risk for heatstroke is a key to prevention. In addition, effective preventive measures include acclimatization to ambient heat and heat conditions, reduction of the extent and duration of physical activity, rescheduling very physical activities, maintaining hydration

Table 4		
Severe complications associated with heatstroke		
Encephalopathy	Rhabdomyolysis	Acute renal failure
Myocardial injury	Hepatocellular injury and failure	Intestinal ischemia
Disseminated intravascular coagulation	Acute respiratory distress syndrome	Pancreatic injury
Blood clots in the stomach and small intestine	Cytoplasmic protein clumping in the spleen	Multiple organ dysfunction

Adapted from Epstein Y, Roberts WO. The pathophysiology of heat stroke: an integrative view of the final common pathway. Scand J Med Sci Sports 2011;21:742–8; with permission.

with nonalcoholic fluids, and removing vulnerable persons at risk from stressful heat environments.[7] The essence of successful resuscitation of heatstroke depends on early recognition and rapid cooling. In the critical care setting, nurses must also be alert to the potential complications related to cellular and organ dysfunction that might have occurred before interventions could be instituted. The earlier an intervention is instituted in the presence of heatstroke, the better the patient's outcome.[14] A list of risk factors for persons prone to heatstroke is presented in **Table 5**.

Once hyperthermia is determined, rapid cooling by any method available reduces the morbidity associated with hyperthermia, and can be life-saving.[33] Although cold-water immersion is the method of choice, this is not always possible. Cold-water immersion is associated with the lowest morbidity and mortality rates. Persons with exertional heatstroke who are treated with immediate immersion have a survival rate of almost 100%.[34,35] Other methods, such as rapidly rotating ice-water–soaked towels or clothing to the head, neck, axilla, and groin, cool-water immersion, or a continuous spray of cold water can be nearly as effective as cold-water immersion.[14,33,34] Some reports advocate the use of iced gastric, bladder, or peritoneal lavage.[36] The overall goal of intervention is to remove as much body heat as rapidly as possible to stop the uncompensated phase of activity and to preserve cellular and organ function.

People who are prone to heatstroke and people who work with persons at risk for heatstroke should be aware of conditions that put them at risk so that immediate and early intervention can be instituted. Despite rapid cooling, there are data identifying that about 30% of heatstroke survivors experience some form of permanent neurologic impairments that are most likely related to cerebellar atrophy and/or infarcts.[37,38] With rapid cooling, most organs that have been compromised by overheated cells can return to normal function if organ perfusion is maintained and cell death is minimized.[39] It has been demonstrated that even though limiting activity in hot-weather conditions can reduce the incidence of heatstroke, exertional heatstroke has been witnessed in even low-risk weather conditions,[39] hence the importance of identification of persons at risk (see **Table 5**).

During the whole intervention, stabilization of patient's airway, breathing, and circulation is paramount. Because of the neurologic consequences associated with heatstroke, these essential functions could experience an interruption at any time. To enhance circulation and protect renal blood flow, to avoid complications such as rhabdomyolysis, intravenous hydration should be instituted as quickly as possible.

Table 5
Risk factors for heatstroke: conditions, characteristics, and occupational risks

Cognitive impairment	Heart and lung diseases	Limited access to air-conditioning
Inner city habitation	Older than 65 y	Younger than 15 y
Living on higher floors in buildings	Persons who must wear protective clothing in hot weather	Persons with skin diseases (eczema, poison ivy, skin graft, burns)
Mental illness	Obesity	Physical disability/impaired mobility
Poor level of fitness	Sickle cell trait	Strenuous exercise during hottest hours
Chronic inflammatory conditions	Athletes	Occupational workers
Military personnel	Farmers	Homeless individuals

Rhabdomyolysis is usually identified through red-brown urine of the patient, and can lead to coagulopathies and death even in patients who are otherwise asymptomatic.[7]

PHARMACOLOGIC INTERVENTIONS

At present, there is little evidence to support the use of anticytokine, antiendotoxin, or anticoagulation therapies in the treatment of heatstroke.[7] Even clinical trials involving sepsis indicate cautious optimism for the use of these therapies. Clinical trials have shown no benefit on overall mortality with sepsis from using antiendotoxin antibodies, ibuprofen, platelet-activating factor receptor antagonists, anti–tumor necrosis factor monoclonal antibodies, or certain interleukins.[7,39] In addition, other nonsteroidal anti-inflammatory drugs, despite their potent anticoagulant and antipyretic effects, have not been tested to determine their efficacy on heatstroke outcomes. Recombinant human activated protein C has potent anticoagulant and antipyretic properties, but before it was tested in heatstroke patients it was removed from the market following revocation of Food and Drug Administration approval.

There are accounts of patients with heatstroke being given dantrolene.[11] This muscle relaxant limits heat generated by muscle activity, which accelerates cooling attempts. In addition, dantrolene attenuates the quantity of calcium released from the sarcoplasmic reticulum of skeletal muscle to cytosol, inhibiting calcium-dependent muscle contraction.[11,40] As a result of this property, calcium-dependent excitation-contraction coupling and muscle contractions are inhibited. Further data are warranted on the use of dantrolene as an adjunctive treatment for heatstroke, and it should not be used independently of other methods of lowering body temperature.

Pharmacologic interventions might be warranted to eliminate the further production of heat from the patient, such as shivering or agitation. These conditions may be treated with benzodiazepines.[41,42] Seizure activity, which also elevates body temperature, should also be treated with benzodiazepines.[41,42] Barbiturates or paralytics alongside intubation and mechanical ventilation are sometimes used for refractory seizures, but evidence indicates that phenytoin is ineffective in seizures related to heat illnesses.

ONGOING INTERVENTIONS

The goal of cooling is to reduce the patient's core temperature to approximately 39°C (102.2°F).[41] The most reliable measures of core body temperature are rectal, or esophageal measurements and core temperatures measured via invasive monitoring apparatus should a device be inserted to measure cardiac parameters. Other measures have been the source of much debate, and are not considered reliable measures of core body temperature. Keeping the goal in mind, it is important not to overcool the patient because this may lead to shivering and, possibly, hypothermia.

The patient's mentation, along with airway and breathing, warrants monitoring. Patients who cannot protect their airway require intubation and mechanical ventilation. Patients who are awake and alert should receive supplemental oxygen.[41] One must keep in mind that even as the temperature of the patient decreases there are several other potential issues that can result from the original heatstroke, as identified in **Table 4**. The critical care nurse must be vigilant for any symptoms or signs that these complications are occurring. The complete focus is therefore not on the patient's temperature alone.

The administration of continuing intravenous fluids depends on the patient's status and underlying conditions, including cardiovascular disease and hypovolemia. Cooling alone often improves cardiac function and hypotension.[42,43]

Other parameters that warrant monitoring include accurate urine output, along with close observance of heart rate and blood pressure. If the patient is not showing improvement over time, a central venous catheter or pulmonary catheter might be required to evaluate hemodynamic parameters and guide administration of fluids. In cases where the central venous pressure is elevated yet the patient continues to be hypotensive, dobutamine is considered the inotrope of choice.[41,42]

SUMMARY

Managing a patient with heatstroke involves assessment and treatment of multiple body systems, as the illness is a systemic disease with high mortality. Critical care is most appropriate for a patient who has endured a heatstroke that is either exertional or classic. Heat-related illnesses that are lower on the continuum can often be treated on site or in an emergency department, where the patient can be released to home, although this would be contingent on other factors such as age, medical condition of the patient, and comorbidities. For example, it would be inappropriate to discharge an elderly, homeless person back to a hot environment with no medical or social support to ameliorate the condition that prompted the visit. Vigilante monitoring of the patient during and after cooling is essential, as the mortality associated with heatstroke is often the result of physiologic processes that have occurred during the hyperthermic episode.

REFERENCES

1. O'Neill MS, Ebi KL. Temperature extremes and health: impacts of climate variability and change in the United States. J Occup Environ Med 2009;51(1):13–25.
2. Centers for Disease Control and Prevention (CDC). Heat-related deaths—United States 1999-2003. MMWR Morb Mortal Wkly Rep 2006;55:796–8.
3. Centers for Disease Control and Prevention (CDC). Heat-related mortality—Arizona 1993-2002. and United States, 1979-2002. MMWR Morb Mortal Wkly Rep 2005;54:628–30.
4. Metzger KB, Ito K, Matte TD. Summer heat and mortality in New York City: how hot is too hot? Environ Health Perspect 2010;118(1):80–5.
5. Gasparrini A, Armstrong B. The impact of heat waves on mortality. Epidemiology 2011;22(1):68–73.
6. Nelson NG, Collins CL, Comstock RD, et al. Exertional heat-related injuries treated in emergency departments in the U.S., 1997-2006. Am J Prev Med 2011;40(1):54–60.
7. Leon LR, Helwig BG. Role of endotoxin and cytokines in the systemic inflammatory response to heat injury. Front Biosci 2010;2:916–38.
8. Howe AS, Boden BP. Heat related illnesses in athletes. Am J Sports Med 2007; 35(8):1384–95.
9. Becker JA, Stewart LK. Heat-related illness. Am Fam Physician 2011;83(11): 1325–30.
10. Winkenwerder W, Sawka M. Disorders due to heat and cold. In: Golman L, editor. Cecil medicine. Philadelphia: Elsevier; 2008.
11. Hashim IA. Clinical biochemistry of hypothermia. Ann Clin Biochem 2010;47: 516–23.
12. Boulant JA. Cellular mechanisms of temperature sensitivity in hypothalamic neurons. Prog Brain Res 1998;115:3–8.
13. Cusack L, Crepigny C, Athanasos P. Heatwaves and their impact on people with alcohol, drug and mental health conditions: a discussion paper on the clinical practice considerations. J Adv Nurs 2011;67(4):915–22.

14. Epstein Y, Roberts WO. The pathophysiology of heat stroke: an integrative view of the final common pathway. Scand J Med Sci Sports 2011;21:742–8.
15. Charkoudian N. Skin blood flow in adults human thermoregulation: how it works, when it does not, and why. Mayo Clin Proc 2003;78:603–12.
16. Gabay C, Kushner I. Acute-phase proteins and other systemic responses to inflammation [Erratum appears in N Engl J Med 1999;340:1376]. N Engl J Med 1999;340:448–54.
17. Bouchama A, Dehbi B, Mohamed G, et al. Prognostic factors in heat waves-related deaths. Arch Intern Med 2007;167:2170–6.
18. Horowitz M. Heat acclimation and cross tolerance against novel stressors: genomic-physiological linkage. Prog Brain Res 2007;162:373–92.
19. Knochel JP, Goodman EL. Heat stroke and other forms of hyperthermia. In: Mackowiak PA, editor. Fever: basic mechanisms and management. Philadelphia: Lippincott-Raven Pub; 1997. p. 437–57.
20. Bouchama A, Knochel JM. Heat stroke. N Engl J Med 2002;346:1978–88.
21. Lambert GP. Role of gastrointestinal permeability in exertional heatstroke. Exerc Sport Sci Rev 2004;32:185–90.
22. Gathiram P, Wells MT, Brock-Utne JG, et al. Portal and systemic arterial plasma lipopolysaccharide concentrations in heat stressed primates. Circ Shock 1988; 25:223–30.
23. Seijo BK, Wielock T. Cerebral metabolism in ischemia: neurochemical basis for therapy. Br J Anaesth 1985;57:47–62.
24. Hubbard RW, Mathew CB, Durkot MJ, et al. Novel approaches to the pathophysiology of heatstroke: the energy depletion model. Ann Emerg Med 1987;16: 1066–75.
25. Hubbard RW. Heatstroke pathophysiology: the energy depletion model. Med Sci Sports Exerc 1990;22:19–28.
26. Yan YE, Zhao YQ, Wang H, et al. Pathophysiological factors underlying heatstroke. Med Hypotheses 2006;67:609–17.
27. Gaffin SL. Simplified calcium transport and storage pathways. J Therm Biol 1999; 24:251–4.
28. Koratich M, Gaffin SL. Mechanisms of calcium transport in human endothelial cells subjected to hyperthermia. J Therm Biol 1999;24:245–9.
29. Gader AM, al-Mashhadani SA, al-Harthy SS. Direct activation of platelets by heat is the possible trigger of the coagulopathy of heat stroke. Br J Haematol 1990;74: 86–92.
30. White JG. Effects of heat on platelet structure and function. Blood 1968;32:324–35.
31. Barbui T, Falanga A. Disseminated intravascular coagulation in acute leukemia. Semin Thromb Hemost 2001;27:593–604.
32. Bouchama A, De Vol AB. Acid-base alterations in heatstroke. Intensive Care Med 2001;27:680–5.
33. Hadad E, Rav-Asha M, Heled Y, et al. Heat stroke: a review of cooling methods. Sports Med 2004;34:501–11.
34. Casa DJ, McDermott BP, Lee EC, et al. Cold water immersion: the gold standard for exertional heat stroke treatment. Exerc Sport Sci Rev 2007;35:141–9.
35. Proulx CI, Ducharme MB, Kenny GP. Effect of water temperature on cooling efficacy during hyperthermia in humans. J Appl Physiol 2003;94(4):1317–23.
36. Smith ME. Cooling treatment of exertional heat illness. Br J Sports Med 2005;39: 503–7.
37. Argaud L, Ferry T, Le QH, et al. Short and long-term outcomes of heatstroke following the 2003 heat wave in Lyon, France. Arch Intern Med 2007;167:2177–83.

38. Dematte JE, O'Mara K, Buescher J, et al. Near-fatal heatstroke during the 1995 heat wave in Chicago. Ann Intern Med 1998;129:173–81.

39. Roberts WO. Exertional heat stroke during a cool weather marathon: a case study. Med Sci Sports Exerc 2006;38:1197–202.

40. Hadad E, Cohen-Sivan Y, Heled Y, et al. Clinical review: treatment of heat stroke: should dantrolene be considered. Crit Care 2005;9(1):86–91.

41. Mattis JG, Yates AM. Heat stroke: helping patients keep their cool. Nurse Pract 2011;36(5):48–52.

42. Helman R, Habal R. Heatstroke. eMedicine; 2009. Available at: http://emedicine.medscape.com/article/166320. Accessed March 20, 2013.

43. Cohen R, Moelleken B. Disorders due to physical agents. In: McPhee SJ, Papadakis MA, Tierney LM, editors. 2007 Current medical diagnosis and treatment. New York: McGraw-Hill Medical; 2007. p. 1624–7.

Hypertrophic Cardiomyopathy
An Overview

K. Melissa Smith, DNP, MSN, ANP-BC*,
Joshua Squiers, PhD, MSN, ANP-BC, AGACNP-BC

KEYWORDS

- Hypertrophic cardiomyopathy • Hypertrophic obstructive cardiomyopathy
- Sudden cardiac death • Left ventricular outflow tract obstruction • Risk stratification
- Sudden death in athletes • Heart failure

KEY POINTS

- Particularly in the summer heat athletes with undiagnosed HCM can experience critical events including sudden cardiac death.
- When histories and physicals result in positive cardiovascular findings, these individuals need referral to cardiovascular specialists.
- Patients with known HCM are also more susceptible to adverse events in the summer months because of the effects of heat and increased activity.
- Patients with HCM may also be admitted to the intensive care unit for other illnesses un-related to HCM.
- The critical care team with deep understanding of the complexities surrounding the diag-nosis and treatment of HCM are better equipped to deliver safe, effective, and excellent care.

INTRODUCTION

Critical care nurses have the responsibility to understand complex cardiovascular disorders. People living with hypertrophic cardiomyopathy (HCM) are particularly susceptible to adverse events when warm weather and strenuous activity are combined. Deeper understanding of the complexity of HCM results in safer bedside care of the patient with HCM who has experienced a critical event. This article reviews the pathophysiology of HCM and the proper screening of athletes for HCM before participation in recreational and competitive sports. Recommendations for activity, symptom management, and current treatment modalities options for patients with HCM are reviewed.

Vanderbilt University School of Nursing, 461 21st avenue, Nashville, TN 37240, USA
* Corresponding author.
E-mail address: k.melissa.smith@vanderbilt.edu

Crit Care Nurs Clin N Am 25 (2013) 263–272
http://dx.doi.org/10.1016/j.ccell.2013.02.011
0899-5885/13/$ – see front matter © 2013 Elsevier Inc. All rights reserved.

INCIDENCE AND PREVALENCE

HCM is a complex, common genetic cardiovascular disease that affects at least 1 in 500 persons of the general population in the United States. This disease of the myocardium can easily remain undetected until the first symptom of sudden cardiac death (SCD). Although many individuals with HCM are minimally affected and have normal life spans, some patients with HCM have significant disease complications resulting in disease progression and premature death.[1–3] The underlying structural cardiac abnormalities found in HCM potentially affect individuals undertaking rigorous activity, such as athletes. In the United States, HCM is responsible for 48% of SCDs of athletes younger than age 35.[4] Overall, the estimated incidence of athletes that die of cardiovascular causes each year is very low; less than 300 per year out of more than 10 million athletes of all ages that participate in organized sports in the United States.[5] Despite this low incidence the impact of the sudden death of a young person can be profound.

PATHOPHYSIOLOGY

HCM is a disease of the myocardium characterized by ventricular hypertrophy, which can be diffusely distributed or localized to a single myocardial segment. There is a dramatic increase in the myocardial tissue with a nondilated ventricular chamber that is in the absence of other cardiac disease.[1,2,6] A comparison of types of cardiomyopathies and differences in the diameter of the ventricle during systole and diastole is displayed in **Fig. 1**. Severe thickening of ventricle wall is evident with HCM. It is distinctive among the cardiomyopathies and clinically presents in infants through the elderly. Although onset of symptoms can occur at any age, typically symptoms begin between the ages of 20 and 40. Symptoms vary but are a result of the following: (1) left ventricular outflow tract (LVOT) obstruction, (2) diastolic dysfunction, (3) myocardial ischemia, and (4) supraventricular and ventricular arrhythmias.[3,7]

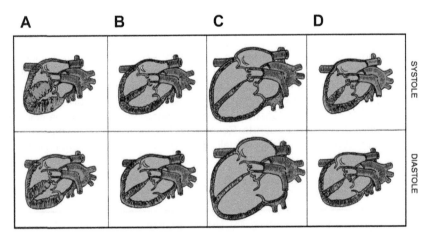

Fig. 1. Types of cardiomyopathies and differences in ventricular diameter during systole and diastole compared with a normal heart. (*A*) Hypertrophic. (*B*) Restrictive. (*C*) Dilated. (*D*) Normal. (*From* Urden LD, Stacy KM, Lough ME. Cardiovascular disorders. In: Urden LD, Stacy KM, Lough ME, editors. Critical care nursing: diagnosis and management. St Louis (MO): Mosby; 2010. p. 466; with permission.)

Left Ventricular Outflow Tract

LVOT obstruction in HCM can be the result of systolic anterior motion of the mitral valve in the presence of septal hypertrophy. This results in mitral-septal contact resulting in partial to complete ventricular outflow obstruction during systole, thus resulting in reserve cardiac flow, subsequent dysrhythmia, and sudden death. Obstruction can also occur from muscular obstruction in the mid cavity region of the LV caused by hypertrophied papillary muscles next to the septum resulting in a functional outflow tract obstruction. Unique to this condition is that the quantity of the LVOT obstruction can change with ventricular cavity size. In particular, reduction of ventricular end diastolic volume, by reduced preload or reduced filling time, can increase the degree of LVOT obstruction.[1,6–8]

Increased myocardial contractility, decreased preload (ie, volume), or decreased after-load (ie, hypotension) can increase the degree of obstruction. Therefore, patients can experience little to no obstruction at rest but generate significant LVOT obstruction with exercise, hypotension, or dehydration.[9] In addition, there is spontaneous variation of the obstruction with changes in day-to-day activities, food and alcohol intake. Symptoms are often exacerbated postprandial and with exercise.[1,6–9] Severity of LVOT obstruction is a major determinant of prognosis and greatly contributes to heart failure–related symptoms that occur in HCM. Additionally, because LVOT can be worsened in the setting of dehydration (reduced preload) and significant tachycardia (reduced filling time), HCM can result in SCD during sports activities.[1–5,7,9–13]

Impact of Diastolic Dysfunction

Diastolic dysfunction is the pathophysiologic process that contributes to most nonobstructive symptoms experienced by the patient with HCM. Because of the hypertrophied cardiac muscle, there can be impaired relaxation of the ventricle resulting in the inability of the chamber to fill rapidly. Abnormal relaxation and filling of the ventricles is present in 80% of patients with HCM.[3] As a result, there is a fine balance for maintaining adequate volume status. Heart failure symptoms occur when there is volume overload in the slow to fill, hypertrophied cardiac muscle of the patient with HCM. Symptoms of pulmonary congestion, such as severe exertional dyspnea, exercise intolerance, and fatigue, are the first symptoms of volume overload to occur. If enough volume overload is present, right-sided symptoms, such as peripheral edema, become apparent.[3] Conversely, patients with HCM with only mild volume depletion are susceptible to significant dizziness, presyncope, and syncope.[1,2,5,9,12]

Angina

Angina is a common symptom of HCM. Although the exact pathophysiologic process is unknown, several processes are thought to contribute to myocardial ischemic in HCM. These include (1) compromised blood flow caused by abnormal intramural coronary arteries, (2) increased myocardial oxygen demand beyond the capacity of the coronary artery system, and (3) diastolic dysfunction resulting in elevated myocardial wall tension.[3,9,14]

Arrhythmia

Arrhythmias are of particular concern for the patient with HCM. Because of the left hypertrophied muscle there is disorganization of cardiac muscle cells, which can impair intercellular transmission along the electrical pathways of the left ventricle (LV). Disorganization of the myocytes predisposes the HCM heart to electrical instability resulting in arrhythmias including exercise-induced tachyarrhythmias. Supraventricular arrhythmias including atrial fibrillation are also very common.[1,2,5,12,15,16]

DEFINITION AND DIFFERENTIAL DIAGNOSIS

HCM is a hereditary genetic disorder of the cardiac sarcomere, and can be defined as unexplained left ventricular hypertrophy with a nondilated ventricular chamber in the absence of other cardiac disease.[1,2,6] If HCM is suspected, a referral to a cardiovascular specialist is imperative because echocardiography is the standard for confirming a diagnosis of HCM.[6] Symptomatic patients with HCM may first present with exercise intolerance, exertional dyspnea, chest pain, palpitations, dizziness, presyncope, and syncope. Most patients with HCM are asymptomatic and live a full life expectancy, although there are cases where the first presentation of HCM is a SCD event.[1,3,10]

Symptoms

Often symptoms of HCM first appear during the adolescent growth period.[6] Patients with symptomatic HCM can present with a variety of clinical symptoms including dyspnea on exertion, fatigue, chest pain, presyncope and syncope, and palpitations. These symptoms can further develop to classic advanced heart failure symptoms, including orthopnea, edema, and paroxysmal nocturnal dyspnea. Dyspnea is the most common symptom found in patients with HCM, and typically results from diastolic dysfunction and poor LV emptying secondary to LVOT obstruction. Any of these cardiac symptoms warrants referral to a clinical provider with expertise in cardiology.[1–5,15,17]

These cardiac findings have a broad differential (eg, idiopathic cardiomyopathy, aortic stenosis, restrictive cardiomyopathy, amyloidosis, and athletic cardiac hypertrophy), but typically echocardiograms should be used for identification of cardiac structural abnormalities including ventricular hypertrophy and LVOT obstruction. In cases where LVOT obstruction is suspected, but the LVOT gradient is less than 50 mm Hg, stress echocardiography should be considered to quantify the potential risk of obstruction. In general, if the left ventricular hypertrophy can be explained by any other disease process, such as long-standing hypertension or infiltrative storage disorders, HCM can be ruled out.[1,7]

After HCM is diagnosed, echocardiograms should be repeated every 12 to 18 months. Twenty-four hour Holter monitoring should be completed every 1 to 2 years to quantify potential risk of dysrhythmia, and identify patients who need referral for further intervention. In cases where a family history is identified, echocardiographic screening of relatives should be considered along with appropriate genetic testing.[1]

Clinical Progression

HCM has three intertwined pathways of clinical progression. Often one or all three of the following occur: (1) SCD caused by unpredictable ventricular tachycardia; (2) progressively worsening heart failure symptoms that include severe dyspnea and angina that eventually leads to end-stage heart failure, and (3) atrial fibrillation that is associated with heart failure with increased risk for thromboembolism and stroke. It is thought that many people have HCM and yet are asymptomatic and achieve a normal life expectancy without any profound complications.[1]

SPORTS PHYSICALS

The importance of a thorough cardiac history and physical examination cannot be underestimated in the sports physical. Any abnormal cardiac finding, or familial history of SCD at less than 35 years of age, warrants referral to a cardiologist for further investigation. Preparticipation sports physical along with appropriate referral remains the best preventative strategy for identification of asymptomatic individuals.[4]

There is precedence for cardiovascular screening of the elite athlete in many collegiate programs and professional athletic programs.[4] Yet, all sports physicals should include a thorough cardiac history and cardiac examination. History questions should include history of murmur, congenital heart defects, family history of heart disease, and family history SCD especially younger than age 35 (**Box 1**). A history of syncope during exercise, external chest pain, or excessive exertional dyspnea should be thoroughly investigated even in younger patients.[4,10]

Physical examination of a patient with HCM may reveal several cardiac abnormalities including split S2, S3 gallop, or a fourth heart sound. Systolic ejection crescendo-decresencdo murmur or holosystolic murmurs may be heard, but are often difficult to detect. Electrocardiogram can provide useful information regarding underlying electrical or structural abnormalities that can place patients at risk, but is not a definitive diagnostic tool for HCM.[4]

ACTIVITY RECOMMENDATIONS

There are approximately 10 to 15 million athletes participating in a broad variety of organized sports in the United States, yet the number of athletes that die from SCD each year is relatively low at less than 300.[5] Physical activities during training or competition seem to trigger most sudden deaths in athletes. Data from the registry of Minneapolis Heart Institute Foundation found that HCM was the cause of SCD in 26.4% of the young athletes studied.[5] The consensus recommendation from the Twenty-sixth Bethesda Conference is that any athlete with probable or conclusive evidence of cardiovascular disease, such as HCM, should be disqualified to participate in sports training and competition.[5]

SCD is not the only concern for patients with HCM participating in activities (recreational or competitive). HCM is considered to be in the category of genetic cardiovascular disease and there are specific exercise recommendations for this category of patients (**Table 1**). Patients with HCM should avoid any sports that include sprinting, such as full-court basketball, soccer, and tennis, but other low-intensity sports that could be dangerous because of loss of consciousness should also be avoided.

Box 1
Example of cardiac history questions for sports physicals

- Have you ever passed out (fainted) while exercising?
- Have you ever had chest pain or chest discomfort while exercising?
- Do you experience shortness of breath during exercise or with minimal activity?
- Has anyone in your family[a] died from a heart problem?
- Does anyone in your family see a specialist for their heart?
- Has anyone in your family died suddenly? If yes, what was the cause of death and their age at death?
- Were you born with any heart problems or defects?
- Have you ever been told you have a heart murmur?

  [a] Include immediate family members and grandparents, aunts, uncles, and cousins.

Table 1
Activity recommendations for the patient with HCM

Recommended	Not Recommended
Lap swimming	Sprinting
Treadmill walking	Basketball
Stationary biking	Tennis
Bowling	Soccer
Golf	Football
Skating	Training for distance road running, biking, or rowing
Snorkeling	Lifting free weights
Non–free weights	Downhill skiing
Brisk walking	Ice hockey
	Rock climbing
	Horseback riding
	Motorcylcing
	Thrill rides (roller coasters)
	Scuba diving
	Platform diving

Data from Maron BJ, Chaitman BR, Ackerman MJ, et al. Recommendations for physical activity and recreational sports participation for young patients with genetic cardiovascular diseases. Circulation 2004;109(22):2807–1.

Exercising in extreme temperatures should definitely be avoided in patients with HCM. Temperatures greater than 80°F or less than 32°F should be avoided, in addition to extreme humidity or high altitudes. Patients with HCM can participate in activities in which energy expenditure is stable and consistent, such as swimming laps or biking on level terrain.[15] Because of the particular risk of decreased preload of the disease process, patients with HCM should take specific measures to stay well hydrated throughout any physically exerting activities. Remaining euvolemic should be a priority for the active patient with HCM.[9,15]

Careful screening of athletes for HCM before participation in high-intensity competitive sports is important and can play a role in prevention of SCD.[1,4] Placement of automatic external defibrillators in schools, athletic settings, sports arenas, and practice areas is evidenced based and highly recommended.[15] It is also particularly important to keep athletes well hydrated because dehydration and HCM is a dangerous combination.[17]

TREATMENT MODALITIES

Treatment of patients with HCM requires a comprehensive understanding of the pathophysiologic complexities and is best managed by clinical providers specializing in cardiovascular care. Treatments must be individualized to the particular presentation of each patient. Many patients who present with HCM are asymptomatic and most achieve normal life expectancies. One goal for asymptomatic patients with HCM is to educate the patient and families that screening of first-degree relatives for HCM should occur.[1,18] When HCM is first found, a SCD risk stratification should be calculated for asymptomatic and symptomatic patients with HCM and should be done by a cardiologist (**Box 2**).[1]

Avoidance of particularly strenuous activities and competitive sports should be emphasized. In addition, avoiding environmental situations where vasodilation may occur should be a priority, as should remaining hydrated.[1] When a patient is known to have HCM but is asymptomatic and requiring treatment of other diseases, such

> **Box 2**
> **SCD risk stratification**
>
> - Personal history of ventricular fibrillation, sustained ventricular tachycardia, or SCD event
> - Presence of an implantable cardiac defibrillator
> - Family history of SCD events or family member with implantable cardiac defibrillator
> - Unexplained syncope
> - Documented nonsustained ventricular tachycardia on Holter monitoring
> - Echocardiographic finding of LV wall thickness greater than or equal to 30 mm.
>
> *Adapted from* Gersh BJ, Maron BJ, Bonow RO, et al. 2011 ACCF/AHA guideline for the diagnosis and treatment of HCM: a report of the American College of Cardiology Foundation/American Heart Association Task Force on Practice Guidelines. J Thorac Cardiovasc Surg 2011;142(6):e153–203; with permission.

as hypertension, it is also important to avoid such medications as high-dose diuretics and vasodilators.[1,3] Advanced therapies, such as septal myectomy or alcohol septal ablation, should not be performed regardless of whether or not LVOT is present.[9]

For symptomatic patients with HCM the treatment goals are directed toward altering the natural course of the disease. Pharmacologic therapy for symptomatic patients can be used to alleviate symptoms of exertional dyspnea, palpitations, and chest discomfort. β-Blockers are the first-line agents because of their negative inotropic properties and ability to slow adrenergic-induced tachycardia.[19] Slowing down the heart rate also improves diastolic filling. Low-dose verapamil if used with caution is effective in providing symptomatic relief for those patients unable to tolerate β-blockers. Verapamil should not be given to patients with systemic hypotension or severe dyspnea at rest.[1] For patients with HCM with LVOT who do not respond to β-blockers or verapamil alone, it is reasonable to combine disopyramide with a β-blocker or verapamil to treat symptoms of angina or dyspnea.[1,6,9] Pure vasoconstricting agents, such as phenylephrine, can be used in cases of obstructive patients with HCM with acute hypotension who do not respond to fluid resuscitation.[1]

Despite good medical therapy, persistent signs and symptoms of volume overload occur. In cases such as these, diuretics are used with extreme caution. Oral loop diuretics, such as furosemide, or thiazide diuretics, such as hydrochlorothiazide, should be used with caution and dosed on an individual basis; the patient should be closely monitored.[9] Overdiuresis of the patient with HCM can result in severe symptoms of volume depletion.[1,6,9] Angiotensin-converting enzyme inhibitors or angiotensin receptor blockers for treatment of symptoms is not well established and should be used with caution.[1] Medications that are contraindicated for patients with HCM include digitalis and dihydropyridine calcium channel blockers, such as nifedipine. Intravenous positive inotropic drugs, such as dopamine, dobutamine, and norephinephrine, are absolutely contraindicated.[1] A summary of pharmacologic therapy is provided in **Table 2**.

INVASIVE THERAPY

Invasive therapies for symptomatic patients with HCM that meet criteria include the following: (1) implantable cardiac defibrillators for secondary or primary prevention of SCD, (2) surgical septal myectomy or alcohol septal ablation for progressive and

Table 2
Pharmacologic therapy for HCM

Safe and Effective	Use with Caution	Contraindicated
β-Blockers: low dose may titrate up to keep resting heart rate 60–65 bpm for persistent dyspnea and angina	β-Blockers: with sinus bradycardia or severe conduction disease	Nifedipine and other dihydropyridine calcium channel blockers
Verapamil: start low dose titrating up to 480 mg/day for persistent dyspnea and angina	Verapamil with advanced heart failure	Digitalis
IV phenylephrine for treatment of acute hypotension, unresponsive to fluid resuscitation	Disopyramide in combination with verapamil or β-blocker	Disopyramide alone
	Loop and thiazide diuretics	IV inotropic medications: dobutamine, milrinone, dopamine, norepinephrine
	Angiotensin-converting enzyme inhibitors, angiotensin receptor blockers	

Data from Gersh BJ, Maron BJ, Bonow RO, et al. 2011 ACCF/AHA guideline for the diagnosis and treatment of hypertrophic cardiomyopathy: a report of the American College of Cardiology Foundation/American Heart Association Task Force on Practice Guidelines. J Thorac Cardiovasc Surg 2011;142(6):e153–203; and Naghi JJ, Siegel RJ. Medical management of hypertrophic cardiomyopathy. Rev Cardiovasc Med 2010;11(4):202–17.

drug-refractory heart failure caused by LVOT obstruction, and (3) heart transplantation for systolic dysfunction with refractory heart failure symptoms. Patients with HCM who develop atrial fibrillation should be treated on an individualized basis, but treatment can include radiofrequency ablation or surgical maze procedure.[1,10,20–22]

SUMMARY

Particularly in the summer heat athletes with undiagnosed HCM can experience critical events including SCD. Because symptoms of HCM often manifest in young adults, it is imperative to perform thorough histories and physicals.[6] When histories and physicals result in positive cardiovascular findings, these individuals need referral to cardiovascular specialists. If patients have relatives with history of sudden death at age 35 or younger, they must be referred for further testing. Patients with known HCM are also more susceptible to adverse events in the summer months because of the effects of heat and increased activity. Often patients with HCM require treatment in the intensive care unit for adverse events directly related to HCM or postoperatively from invasive treatments. Patients with HCM may also be admitted to the intensive care unit for other illnesses unrelated to HCM. Regardless of the reason for admission to the critical care unit, the patient with a history of HCM needs special considerations. The critical care team with deep understanding of the complexities surrounding the diagnosis and treatment of HCM is better equipped to deliver safe, effective, and excellent care. With proper care and caution, persons with HCM can live long and productive lives.

REFERENCES

1. Gersh BJ, Maron BJ, Bonow RO, et al. 2011 ACCF/AHA guideline for the diagnosis and treatment of hypertrophic cardiomyopathy: a report of the American College of Cardiology Foundation/American Heart Association Task Force on Practice Guidelines. J Thorac Cardiovasc Surg 2011;142(6):e153–203.
2. Graham-Cryan MA, Rowe G, Hathaway L, et al. Obstructive hypertrophic cardiomyopathy. Prog Cardiovasc Nurs 2004;19(4):133–40.
3. Fuster VA, Alexander RW, O'Rourke RA, editors. Hurst's the heart. 10th edition. New York: McGraw-Hill Medical Publishing Division; 2001.
4. Battle RW, Mistry DJ, Malhotra R, et al. Cardiovascular screening and the elite athlete: advances, concepts, controversies, and a view of the future. Clin Sports Med 2011;30(3):503–24.
5. Maron BJ, Zipes DP. Introduction: eligibility recommendations for competitive athletes with cardiovascular abnormalities—general considerations. J Am Coll Cardiol 2005;45(8):1318–21.
6. Naghi JJ, Siegel RJ. Medical management of hypertrophic cardiomyopathy. Rev Cardiovasc Med 2010;11(4):202–17.
7. Maron MS, Olivotto I, Zenovich AG, et al. Hypertrophic cardiomyopathy is predominantly a disease of left ventricular outflow tract obstruction. Circulation 2006;114(21):2232–9.
8. Geske JB, Sorajja P, Ommen SR, et al. Left ventricular outflow tract gradient variability in hypertrophic cardiomyopathy. Clin Cardiol 2009;32(7):397–402.
9. Fifer MA, Vlahakes GJ. Management of symptoms in hypertrophic cardiomyopathy. Circulation 2008;117(3):429–39.
10. Maron BJ. Sudden death in young athletes. N Engl J Med 2003;349(11):1064–75.
11. Kansal MM, Mookadam F, Tajik AJ. Drink more, and eat less: advice in obstructive hypertrophic cardiomyopathy. Am J Cardiol 2010;106(9):1313–6.
12. Link MS, Estes NA. Sudden cardiac death in athletes. Prog Cardiovasc Dis 2008; 51(1):44–57.
13. Sorajja P, Allison T, Hayes C, et al. Prognostic utility of metabolic exercise testing in minimally symptomatic patients with obstructive hypertrophic cardiomyopathy. Am J Cardiol 2012;109(10):1494–8.
14. Lele SS, Thomson HL, Seo H, et al. Exercise capacity in hypertrophic cardiomyopathy. Role of stroke volume limitation, heart rate, and diastolic filling characteristics. Circulation 1995;92(10):2886–94.
15. Rothmier JD, Drezner JA. The role of automated external defibrillators in athletics. Sports Health 2009;1(1):16–20.
16. Maron BJ, Shen WK, Link MS, et al. Efficacy of implantable cardioverter-defibrillators for the prevention of sudden death in patients with hypertrophic cardiomyopathy. N Engl J Med 2000;342(6):365–73.
17. Maron BJ, Chaitman BR, Ackerman MJ, et al. Recommendations for physical activity and recreational sports participation for young patients with genetic cardiovascular diseases. Circulation 2004;109(22):2807–16.
18. Spirito P, Seidman CE, McKenna WJ, et al. The management of hypertrophic cardiomyopathy. N Engl J Med 1997;336(11):775–85.
19. Cecchi F, Olivotto I, Gistri R, et al. Coronary microvascular dysfunction and prognosis in hypertrophic cardiomyopathy. N Engl J Med 2003;349(11): 1027–35.
20. Sorajja P, Valeti U, Nishimura RA, et al. Outcome of alcohol septal ablation for obstructive hypertrophic cardiomyopathy. Circulation 2008;118(2):131–9.

21. Harris KM, Spirito P, Maron MS, et al. Prevalence, clinical profile, and significance of left ventricular remodeling in the end-stage phase of hypertrophic cardiomyopathy. Circulation 2006;114(3):216–25.
22. Callans DJ. Ablation of atrial fibrillation in the setting of hypertrophic cardiomyopathy. J Cardiovasc Electrophysiol 2008;19(10):1015–6.

Burns

Deborah L. Ellison, PhD(c), MSN, RN

KEYWORDS

- Burns • Smoke inhalation • Carbon monoxide • Fluid resuscitation
- Burn wound sepsis

KEY POINTS

- Over the past 2 decades there has been significant decline in the number of burn injuries, hospitalizations, and deaths caused by burns; an acute burn injury remains the third leading cause of death in children between the ages of 1 and 9 years, and it has decreased to the sixth leading cause of death in the rest of the population.
- Burn injuries are described in terms of causative agents, depth, and severity.
- Early fluid resuscitation management is essential to reduce patient mortality and morbidity.
- Concomitant problems encountered in the intensive care units or burn units include inhalation injury, carbon monoxide toxicity and cyanide poisoning, and burn wound sepsis.
- Critical care nursing is interprofessional, supportive, and preventive management.

INTRODUCTION

Summer is a time of increased activity, but this carries risks. Summer activities such as barbecuing, camping, and fireworks happen all over the country, but can be dangerous for potential burns. A burn is defined as a traumatic injury to the skin or other organic tissue primarily caused by thermal or other acute exposure.[1] In the past 2 decades there has been a significant decline in the number of burn injuries, hospitalizations, and deaths, but an acute burn injury remains the third leading cause of death in children between the ages of 1 and 9 years, and it has decreased to the sixth leading cause of death in the remaining population.[2]

The American Burn Association statistics from 2001 to 2010 for admissions to burn centers are as follows:

- Survival rate: 96.1%
- Gender: 70% male, 30% female
- Ethnicity: 60% white, 19% African American, 15% Hispanic, 6% other
- Admission cause: 44% fire/flame, 33% scald, 9% contact, 4% electrical, 3% chemical, 7% other
- Place of occurrence: 68% home, 10% occupational, 7% street/highway, 15% other[3]

Austin Peay State University, PO Box 4658, 751 York Road, Clarksville, TN 37044, USA
E-mail address: ellisond@apsu.edu

Crit Care Nurs Clin N Am 25 (2013) 273–285
http://dx.doi.org/10.1016/j.ccell.2013.02.003
0899-5885/13/$ – see front matter © 2013 Elsevier Inc. All rights reserved.

ccnursing.theclinics.com

Once a burn patient reaches a local hospital emergency room, patients must initially be treated and then evaluated for transfer to a burn center based on the Burn Center Referral Criteria. A burn center may treat adults, children, or both. The American Burn Association recommendation for referral to a burn center includes:

- Partial-thickness burns greater than 10% of total body surface area (TBSA).
- Burns that involve the face, hands, feet, genitalia, perineum, or major joints.
- Third-degree burns of any age group.
- Electrical burns, including lightning injury.
- Chemical burns.
- Inhalation injury.
- Burn injury in patients with preexisting medical disorders that could complicate management, prolong recovery, or affect mortality.
- Any patient with burns and concomitant trauma (such as fractures) in which the burn injury poses the greatest risk of morbidity or mortality. In such cases, if the trauma poses the greater immediate risk, the patient may initially be stabilized in a trauma center before being transferred to a burn unit. Physician judgment is necessary in such situations and should be in concert with the regional medical control plan and triage protocols.
- Burned children in hospitals without qualified personnel or equipment for the care of children.
- Burn injury in patients who require special social, emotional, or rehabilitative intervention.[2,4]

A patient with a 78% TBSA burn has a 50% chance of survival.[2] Burn centers and the advocacy of national organizations have assisted with the decrease of burns and deaths from burns by increasing fire-resistant products, fire prevention programs, and legislation.[1]

TYPES OF BURN INJURIES

Burn injuries are described in terms of causative agents, depth, and severity.

Causative Agents

Causative agents include thermal burns, chemical burns, and electrical burns. Summer celebrations bring many burn dangers to children, adults, and the elderly. Electrical storms, grills, house fires, explosions, and fireworks are a few of the causes of summer burns.

Thermal burns account for 70% of all burn injuries.[2,5] Some of the most common thermal burns are associated with flame sources such as a house fire, cooking accidents, or a fiery explosion. Scald burns from steam or contact with a hot object, such as a cooking pan or hot steel, may also cause thermal injury.[2,5,6]

Chemical burns are commonly encountered after exposure to acids and alkali. Contact with acid produces tissue coagulation, whereas alkaline burns generate colliquation necrosis.[6] Hydrofluoric acid, formic acid, and anhydrous ammonia are organic compounds included as chemical agents.[2] Other chemical agents that cause chemical burns include white phosphorus, certain elemental metals, nitrates, and hydrocarbons.[2,5] Whatever the agent, contact time is critical in determining the severity of injury and/or life-threatening conditions.[2,3,6]

Electrical burns are the effects of electricity on the body, and happen when electrical energy is transformed into thermal injury as the current passes through poorly conducting body tissues. Five types of assessments are needed for electrical burns: the type of current (alternating or direct), the pathway of the current, the duration of contact, the resistance of the body tissue, and the voltage.[2,3,6]

Depth of Burn

Many factors alter the response of body tissues. The degree or depth of a burn depends on the temperature of the injuring agent, the duration of exposure to the injury agent, and the areas of the body that are exposed to the injuring agent.[2,3,6] The traditional classification of burns as first, second, third, or fourth degree has been replaced by a system reflecting the need for surgical intervention.[6] Damage to the skin is currently defined in terms of superficial, superficial partial thickness, deep partial thickness, and full thickness, which correspond with the various layers of the skin. Fourth degree is used for those burns that extend into the muscle and/or bone.[6] **Table 1** shows the classification of burns, the tissues involved, and the usual causes.

PATHOPHYSIOLOGY

Burns have both a localized tissue response and a systemic response (**Fig. 1**). In the localized tissue response, the cellular injury starts when tissues are exposed to energy sources (thermal, chemical, electrical, or radiation). The depth of the thermal injury is shown by the extent of injury down through the layers of skin. The zone of coagulation is the area where the most damage has been sustained; temperatures have reached 45°C (113° Fahrenheit).[2,5] In this zone of coagulation the tissues are black, gray, khaki, or white.[2,5] The area has lost the ability to recover and requires surgical intervention. This area contains cells that are at most risk during burn resuscitation.[2] They can recover or become necrotic in the initial 24 to 72 hours, depending on the conditions and course of resuscitation. The zone of hyperemia is the area of increased blood flow in order to bring needed nutrients to the tissue for recovery (active hyperemia) and to

Table 1
Classification of burns by depth of injury

Depth	Tissues Involved	Usual Cause	Characteristics
Superficial (first degree)	Epidermis, minimal epithelial damage	Sunburn or brief exposure to hot liquid, flash, flame	Dry, blisters after 24 h, pinkish red, blanches with pressure
Superficial partial thickness (second degree)	Epidermis, superficial dermis	Flash, hot liquids	Moist, pinkish or mottled red, blisters within 24 h, some blanching
Deep partial thickness (second degree)	Epidermis, part of dermis: epidermal-lined hair and sweat glands intact; hair follicles and glandular tissue damaged	Flash, hot liquids, hot solids, flame, and intense radiant injury	Pale/patchy cheesy white to red; wet or waxy dry; almost always blisters; no blanching
Full thickness (third degree)	Epidermis and all layers of the dermis; may involve subcutaneous fat, muscle, and bone	Sustained flame, electrical, chemical, and steam	Can be leathery, cracked, waxy white, cherry red, brown, or black; no blanching; no blisters

Data from Refs.[1,2,6,7]

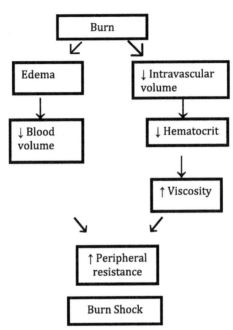

Fig. 1. Pathophysiology map. (*From* Lewis, Dirksen, Heitkemper, et al. Burns. In: Medical surgical nursing: assessment and management of clinical problems. St Louis (MO): Elsevier Mosby; 2011. p. 472–94; with permission.)

remove the metabolic waste products (reactive hyperemia).[2] This area heals rapidly and has no cell death.

Major changes at the cellular level are responsible for the large systemic response noted in a patient with burns. The localized response causes a coagulation of cellular proteins, leading to irreversible cell injury with local production of complement, histamine, and oxygen free radicals (ie, by-products of oxidative processes).[2,5,7] Oxygen free radicals alter cell lipids and proteins, affecting the integrity of the cell membrane, which is particularly problematic in the endothelium of the microvascular circulation because disruption of the cell membrane leads to increased vascular permeability.[2,5,7] Increased vascular permeability leads to loss of plasma proteins into the interstitium and results in a marked decrease in circulation volume. Complement activation and histamine release contribute to the increased vascular permeability by increasing production of oxygen free radicals. Increased vascular permeability leads to the formation of interstitial edema, which usually peaks within 24 to 48 hours of injury.[2,5] The pulmonary interstitial edema forms, with intra-alveolar hemorrhages; this initial insult is thought to be a precursor to the development of acute respiratory distress syndrome (ARDS).[2,5,7]

The systemic response to a burn injury involves the release of vasoactive substances, such as histamine, prostaglandins, interleukins, and arachidonic acid metabolites.[2,5,7] These substances initiate the systemic inflammatory response syndrome (SIRS). The potent mediators and cytokines (nitric oxide, platelet-activating factor, serotonin, thromboxane A_2, and tumor necrosis factor) deplete the intravascular volume, decreasing the blood flow to the kidneys and the gastrointestinal tract.[2,5] If left uncorrected, hypovolemic shock, metabolic acidosis, and hyperkalemia may occur. Intestinal mucosal permeability also markedly increases and can become the primary source of bacterial infection.[2,5,7] Early enteral feeding is one step to help prevent the translocation of bacteria.

RESUSCITATION PHASE

Early management is essential to reduce patient mortality and morbidity. Immediate care involves accurate assessment of burn depth and appropriate fluid management.[8] The main aim of burn care is to restore form, function, and feeling to burn-injured skin to maximize the patient's abilities and promote physical, psychological, and emotional recovery.[8]

Burn shock occurs during the initial 24 to 48 hours following major burns. It is characterized by myocardial depression and increased capillary permeability, resulting in large fluid shifts and depletion of intravascular volume.[6] Therapy for burn shock is designed to support the patient through the hypovolemic shock until capillary integrity is restored.[2,5] The goal of fluid resuscitation is to support end-organ function and perfusion with the smallest amount of fluid possible.[2,9] Fluid therapy must be tailored to each patient in the intensive care unit, while providing hemodynamic stability.[9] Delays in fluid resuscitation are associated with increased mortality. Therefore, even if a patient is transferred to a burn center, fluid resuscitation must begin immediately. According to the American Burn Association's practice guidelines, any patient with greater than 15% TBSA nonsuperficial burns should receive formal fluid resuscitation.[2,5,7] There are 4 goals of fluid resuscitation:

- Correct fluid, electrolyte, and protein deficits
- Replace continuing losses and maintain fluid balance
- Prevent excessive edema formation
- Maintain an hourly urinary output in adults of 30 to 50 mL/h (approximately 0.5 mL/kg/h)[2,5]

One of the most expeditious methods to estimate the TBSA for adults is the Rule of Nines. Using the following percentages, the TBSA can be calculated using the Rule of Nines:

- Each leg represents 18%
- Each arm represents 9%
- The anterior and posterior trunk each represents 18%
- The head represents 9%
- The genital area represents 1%[1,2,5,7]

Several methods have been developed for fluid resuscitation (**Table 2**). They all have advantages and disadvantages, but the American Burn Association recommends a combination of the modified Brooke formula and the Baxter (commonly call the Parkland) formula.[2,5,7] This consensus formula calls for 2 to 4 mL of lactated Ringer solution per kilogram of body weight per percentage of TBSA burn.[2,5,7] The total amount calculated is administered in the first 8 hours from the time of the burn, then one-fourth is given during the next 8 hours, and the remaining one-fourth is given over the next 8 hours.[2,5,7] This is a general formula, and individuals may need more or less than the amount calculated. The challenge is to balance the fluid resuscitation because too little or too much resuscitation have significant consequences to the patient.[1] Avoiding fluid overload and pulmonary edema is difficult with the large amounts of fluid that must be given in the first 24 hours.[1-3,5,7] In general, patients who often require more fluid are those individuals with electrical burns, inhalation injuries, delayed resuscitation, prior dehydration at the time of the injuries, and concomitant trauma.[2,5]

Table 2
Critical care nursing plan of care for fluids/electrolytes

Problem	Interventions
Restoring and maintaining fluid balance Urine output 30–70 mL/h or 0.5 mL/kg/h Central venous pressure 8–12 mm Hg; PAOP 12–18 mm Hg; blood pressure within normal limits (for specific patient); heart rate 100–120 bpm (or WNL for specific patient)	Assess intake and output every 1 h Give lactated Ringer 2–4 mL/kg/TBAS%, divided into first 24-h after the burn (calculated from the time of the burn) Monitor for spontaneous diuresis (a hallmark indicating the end of the resuscitative phase) and reduce intravenous infusion rate as indicated Daily weight Maintain 4 goals in fluid resuscitation Monitor urine output every 1 h (urine output is the single best indicator of fluid)
Electrolytes, mineral and renal function values are within normal limits	Monitor and replace minerals and electrolytes Monitor blood urea nitrogen, creatinine, myoglobin, and urine electrolytes and glucose Monitor neurologic status Monitor and treat dysrhythmias Monitor and limit water consumption; patients with burns have extreme thirst and, if allowed, have greatly decreased sodium levels

Abbreviation: WNL, within normal limits.
Data from Morton P, Fontaine D. Critical care nursing: a holistic approach. 10th edition. Philadelphia: Lippincott William & Wilkins; 2009. p. 1349–73; and Lewis, Dirksen, Heitkemper, et al. Burns. In: Medical surgical nursing: assessment and management of clinical problems. St Louis (MO): Elsevier Mosby; 2011. p. 472–94.

Lactated Ringer solution is the crystalloid of choice for fluid resuscitation because it is a balanced salt solution that closely approximates the composition of extracellular fluid.[2,5] Colloids can be added between 12 and 14 hours, because this is the time in which most patients' capillary integrity is restored.[2,5] Adding the colloids assists in restoring albumin levels to 2 to 3 mg/dL. After the first 24 hours of injury, replacing the massive evaporative water loss is a major consideration in fluid management.[2,5] The primary solution administered at this time is 5% dextrose in water (D_5W), with the goal of keeping the patient's sodium concentration at140 mEq/L.[2]

Urine output is the single best indicator of fluid resuscitation in patients with previously normal renal function.[1,5,6] The onset of spontaneous diuresis is a hallmark indicating the end of the resuscitative phase.[5,6] At this time the infusion rates can be decreased by 20% to 30% for 1 hour and, if the urine output is maintained, then the procedure can be repeated.[1,2,5] It is essential that the hourly urine output in adults be maintained at 30 to 50 mL/h (approximately 0.5 mL/kg/h).[3,5]

CONCOMITANT PROBLEMS

Concomitant problems may be encountered in intensive care units or burn units. Inhalation injury, carbon monoxide toxicity and cyanide poisoning, and burn wound sepsis are the major concomitant problems. Both inhalation injury and carbon monoxide toxicity produce thermal injuries to the airway. Pulmonary damage usually occurs within 24 to 48 hours of the injury and may be secondary to the inhalation of combustible products or the result of inhaled superheated air.[2] Any of the concomitant problems discussed can rapidly change and progress to SIRS, ARDS, and death.

Inhalation Injury

Smoke inhalation is the leading cause of death caused by fires in adults with burns.[6,10] Costs for treating burns resulting from fire/flames are greater than for burns from scalds or contact with hot object.[11] Life lost and duration of hospital stay are greater when a burn is complicated by smoke inhalation.[11] Smoke inhalation causes 3 types of injuries to the lungs and airway: thermal injury to the upper airways, chemical injury to the tracheobronchial tree, and systemic poisoning caused by carbon monoxide and/or cyanide.[10] Therefore, it is critical that the airway is assessed, because airway edema related to a burn can occur rapidly.[6] The clinical manifestations, evaluation, and management of smoke inhalation are discussed later. The initial management of a patient presenting with smoke inhalation is the immediate assessment of the patient's airway, breathing, and circulation as indicated.[6] This initial assessment should only take a few seconds to perform. Goals of successful treatment of inhalation injury include improving oxygenation and decreasing interstitial edema and airway occlusion.[2] Intubation is indicated if any of the following signs and symptoms is present:

- History of incident occurring in a confined area
- Singed nasal or facial hairs
- Burns in the oral or pharyngeal mucous membranes
- Burns in the perioral area or neck
- Carbonaceous sputum
- Change in voice (especially hoarseness)
- Change in level of consciousness
- Persistent cough, stridor, or wheezing
- Deep facial or circumferential neck burns
- Respiratory distress
- Signs and symptoms of hypercapnia or hypoxia
- Increased carbon monoxide and/or cyanide levels[5–7]

If these findings are absent, the oropharynx should be examined, followed by laryngoscopy if there is edema. A bronchoscopy should be performed (instead of a laryngoscopy) if there is a history of inhalation of superheated particles or steam, because thermal injury may involve the lower respiratory tract. The objective of ventilator support is to provide adequate gas exchange at the lowest possible inspired oxygen concentration and airway pressure, in attempt to reduce the incidence of oxygen toxicity and pulmonary barotrauma.[2,5] Instituting a low tidal volume is necessary to minimize airway pressure, which reduces ventilator-associated lung injury and improves outcomes.[6] The following diagnostic examinations assist in the diagnosis and treatment of smoke inhalation:

- Fiberoptic bronchoscopy is used to investigate suspected smoke inhalation and damage from noxious gases. A normal finding includes a normal larynx, trachea, and bronchi. An abnormal finding includes thermal injury and edema to the oropharynx and glottis.[12]
- Carbon monoxide binds to hemoglobin with an affinity 240 times greater than that of oxygen. Carboxyhemoglobin normal levels are 8% to 10% in smokers and less than 8% in nonsmokers; greater than 10% indicates potential inhalation injury and greater than 30% is associated with mental status changes, whereas greater than 60% is lethal.[12]

- Chest radiography should show a normal chest. Abnormal indications include aspiration and pulmonary infiltrates. Chest radiography is a poor predictor of inhalation because of low sensitivity. If infiltrates are shown on the initial evaluation, this could indicate severe injury or a poor prognosis.[6]

Patients who do not require intubation should receive supplemental oxygen at a fraction of inspired oxygen of 100%. Exceptions to 100% oxygen may be patients with a history of chronic obstructive pulmonary disease (COPD) with carbon dioxide retention. The purpose of the high concentration of supplemental oxygen is to quickly reverse tissue hypoxia and to displace carbon monoxide and cyanide from protein-binding sites.[7] Interventions for patients who do not require intubation include high Fowler position, frequent pulmonary toilet, chest physiotherapy, repositioning, cough and deep breathing, and administering aerosolized racemic epinephrine, which may be sufficient to limit further complications.[2]

Carbon Monoxide and Cyanide

Carbon monoxide poisoning should be presumed in all patients who present following smoke inhalation until it is excluded by a normal carboxyhemoglobin level. Normal levels for carboxyhemoglobin level are discussed in **Table 3**. Carboxyhemoglobin levels should be obtained all patients, even if they do not manifest the usual findings of headache, nausea, malaise, altered cognition, dyspnea, angina, seizures, coma, cardiac dysrhythmias, heart failure, and bright cherry-red lips or skin. Bright cherry-red lips and/or skin indicate acute exposure.[2,6,7,12] The initial approach to presumed carbon monoxide poisoning involves administering supplemental oxygen at 100%, following assessment of whether hyperbaric oxygen is indicated.[2,12] Standard pulse oximetry is not reliable with significant carbon monoxide toxicity.[1] The purpose of both supplemental oxygen and hyperbaric oxygen is to displace carbon monoxide from hemoglobin and other proteins, after which it can be expelled through the lungs.[1,2] The hyperbaric oxygen is thought to decrease the half-life of the carboxyhemoglobin by approximately 20 minutes and decrease the incidence of neuropsychological abnormalities.[2]

Hydrogen cyanide is a by-product of the burning of certain compounds. These compounds include polyurethane, acrylonitrile, nylon, wool, and cotton.[10] Hydrogen cyanide inhibits aerobic metabolism and can rapidly result in death.[2] Cyanide poisoning is nearly impossible to confirm during the initial hours following smoke inhalation because cyanide levels cannot be measured soon enough to be clinically useful (**Table 4**).[10] The signs and symptoms of cyanide poisoning include coma, central apnea, cardiac dysfunction, severe lactic acidosis, high mixed venous oxygen, and low arteriovenous O_2 content differences but are nonspecific and may be caused

Table 3 Signs and symptoms of carbon monoxide poisoning	
Carboxyhemoglobin Saturation (%)	Clinical Presentation
10	No symptoms
20	Headache, nausea/vomiting, dyspnea on exertion
30	Confusion, lethargy, tachypnea
40–60	Seizure, coma, change in electrocardiogram
>60	Death

Data from Morton P, Fontaine D. Critical care nursing: a holistic approach. 10th edition. Philadelphia: Lippincott William & Wilkins; 2009. p. 1349–73.

Table 4
Critical care nursing plan of care for inhalation/ventilation

Problem	Intervention
Oxygenation/ventilation	Auscultate breath sounds every 2–4 h and PRN
	Assess for inhalation injury, and anticipate intubation
	Assess endotracheal tube size and placement
	Assess quantity and color of tracheal secretions
	Suction endotracheal airway when needed
	Hyperoxygenate and hyperventilate before and after each suction
	Monitor airway pressures every 1 h
	Monitor lung compliance every 8 h
	Administer bronchodilators and mucolytics as ordered (working with respiratory therapy)
	Perform chest physiotherapy every 4 h
	Monitor airway pressures and lung compliance for improvement after interventions
	Monitor Pao_2/Fio_2 ratio and oxygen index, monitoring trends
	Turn side to side every 2 h
	Consider kinetic therapy or prone positioning
	Daily chest radiograph
	Daily laboratory values as indicated and/or ordered
	Monitor for the progression to ARDS
	Initial and serial carboxyhemoglobin levels until <10%
	Monitor ABGs, acid-base balance, and lactate and bicarbonate levels (Pulse oximetry and calculated Sao_2 are inaccurate measurements in the presence of carbon monoxide)
	Provide humidified oxygen
	Consider hyperbaric therapy

Data from Morton P, Fontaine D. Critical care nursing: a holistic approach. 10th edition. Philadelphia: Lippincott William & Wilkins; 2009. p. 1349–73; and Morton PG, Fontaine DK. Essentials of critical care nursing: a holistic approach. Philadelphia: Lippincott Williams & Wilkins; 2013. p. 1184–208.

by carbon monoxide poisoning or a different inhaled toxin.[2,6] A lactate level greater than or equal to 10 mmol/L is both sensitive and specific for cyanide toxicity in patients with smoke inhalation. A low $Paco_2$ reflects respiratory compensation for the lactic acidosis. Sodium thiosulfate should be initiated with any patient with an unexplained lactic acidosis, low $Paco_2$, or declining $Paco_2$.[10]

Burn Wound Sepsis

An intact, healthy skin surface has bacteriostatic properties that normally limit the degree to which skin is protected from bacteria. Patients with burn injuries lose their protective primary barrier (skin) to environmental microorganisms. The burn consists of avascular necrotic tissue (eschar) that provides a protein-rich environment favorable to microbial colonization (**Table 5**).[13] Vascular collapse from the burn shock is a critical component of the pathophysiologic response to severe burns.[6] Any patient who sustains a severe burn (greater than 20% TBSA) is at a high risk of developing an invasive wound infection, also referred to as burn wound sepsis, which often leads to multiorgan dysfunction and death.[10] The definition of sepsis is complicated in a patient with a burn, because the basic definition for patients without burns does not apply to the severely burned because of the inflammatory mediators that alter the postburn baseline metabolic profiles.[10] The burn sepsis definition distinguishes

Table 5	
Critical care nursing plan of care for infection	
Problem	**Intervention**
Infection	All catheters invading the body, including endotracheal tubes, central venous catheters, and bladder catheters must be strict sterile procedures
	Meticulous washing hands before and after handling the patient, or any item in the room (decreasing colonization of bacteria number 1 intervention)
	Monitor for s/s of sepsis following The American Burn Association definition of sepsis and infection (listed earlier)
	Education of family and friends regarding infection protocols and dangers to patient
	Obtain and monitor quantitative wound cultures
	Obtain and monitor vital signs for s/s of shock

Data from Morton P, Fontaine D. Critical care nursing: a holistic approach. 10th edition. Philadelphia: Lippincott William & Wilkins; 2009. p. 1349–73; and Morton PG, Fontaine DK. Essentials of critical care nursing: a holistic approach. Philadelphia: Lippincott Williams & Wilkins; 2013. p. 1184–208.

the change in the patient status as a result of a microbial infection from changes that happen secondary to the hypermetabolic response of the burn.[13] The classification categories of burn wound infections are bacterial colonization, noninvasive bacterial infection, burn-related surgical wound infection, burn wound cellulitis, burn wound impetigo, and invasive burn infection.[13]

- "A noninvasive bacterial infection in the burn wound and eschar is defined as greater than 10^5 bacteria per gram of tissue. An invasive burn wound infection, also called burn wound sepsis, and is defined as the presence of microorganisms in adjacent unburned tissue. Quantitative burn wound cultures and burn wound histopathology are required to establish the diagnosis of a bacterial infection." (Gauglitz and Shahrokhi[13]). Acute infections manifest as erythema, pain, purulent exudate, and edema surrounding the wound without the systemic findings described in an invasive wound.[13]
- Invasive burn wound infections (greater than 10^5 bacteria per gram of tissue) occur in an unexcised deep partial-thickness or full-thickness burn wound and adjacent unburned tissue.[13]

THE AMERICAN BURN ASSOCIATION DEFINITION OF SEPSIS, INFECTION, AND DOCUMENTATION

The American Burn Association definition of sepsis and infection in burn patients includes at least 3 of the following parameters:

- Temperature greater than 39°C (102.2°F) or less than 36.5°C (97.7°F)
- Progressive tachycardia (more than age-specific normal values)
- Progressive tachypnea (adults: >30 breaths per minute or more than age-specific normal values)
- Refractory hypotension (adults: systolic blood pressure <90 mm Hg or a decrease >40 mm Hg, or a mean atrial pressure <70 mm Hg)
- Leukocytosis (adults: >12,000 white cells/μL)
- Thrombocytopenia that occurs 3 days after resuscitation (adults: <100,000 platelets per μL)
- Hyperglycemia (>110 mg/dL) in the absence of preexisting diabetes mellitus

- Inability to tolerate enteral feedings for more than 24 hours based on abdominal distention, residual volumes (adults: 2 times the feeding rate), and uncontrollable diarrhea (adults: >2500 mL/d)[13]

The American Burn Association requires that the infection be documented by one of the following evaluations.

- Infection confirmed on a culture (wound, blood, or urine), or
- Pathologic tissue source is identified (10^5 bacteria on quantitative wound tissue biopsy or microbial invasion on biopsy), or
- A documented clinical response to antimicrobial administration[13]

Acute Compartment Syndrome

Trauma injuries are often associated with burns. Many patients with burns sustain falls, crushing injuries, or penetrating wounds from the same incidents and these additional injuries contribute to increased compartment syndrome. For acute compartment syndrome, failure to recognize and decompress the muscular compartments in a timely fashion can compromise the extremity or the patient's life.[14] Burns often require decompressive therapies such as escharotomy, fasciotomy, and amputations because of a pathologic process that results in increased pressure of the tissue. In people with burns this may be caused by the massive fluid resuscitation that is required, which can increase pressure in the muscle compartment, or the result of formation of circumferential eschar.[12,14]

- Escharotomy relieves the pressure and restores perfusion to the area by releasing the constricting eschar.[7,12] Escharotomy can be performed anywhere on the body. In general, escharotomies are performed at the bedside in the critical care setting.
- Fasciotomy relieves the pressure and restores perfusion to the area, but the cut is deeper than the escharotomy and goes into the muscle.[7,12] Indications for a fasciotomy include:
  o Failure of escharotomies to restore perfusion
  o Compartment pressure exceeding 30 mm Hg
  o Compartment pressure within 10 to 20 mm Hg of diastolic pressure
  o Decrease in peripheral pulse oximetry to 90%
  o High-voltage (>1000 V) electrical injury[14]
  In general, a fasciotomy is performed in the operating room. However, sometimes a critically ill patient is too unstable to be transported and requires the fasciotomy to be performed at the bedside in the critical care area.[14] In these circumstances, local anesthesia and conscious sedation at a minimum are required.[14]
- Amputations are indicated in cases of severe vascular, tendon, bone, or joint damage.[12]

SUMMARY

Patients with burns require an interprofessional approach in assessment, treatment, and at all recovery stages. Collaboration from team to team, if transferred, and collaboration within each setting is imperative for optimal outcomes for a patient with a burn. Burn injuries are described in terms of causative agents, depth, and severity. **Table 6** shows the classification of burns, the tissues involved, usual causes, characteristics, pain, and healing time.

Table 6
Burn summary highlights

Depth	Tissues Involved	Usual Cause	Characteristics	Pain	Healing
Superficial (first degree)	Epidermis, minimal epithelial damage	Sunburn or brief exposure to hot liquid, flash, flame	Dry, blisters after 24 h, pinkish red, blanches with pressure	Painful, pruritus during healing	3–6 d, no scarring
Superficial partial thickness (second degree)	Epidermis, superficial dermis	Flash, hot liquids	Moist, pinkish or mottled red, blisters within 24 h, some blanching	Pain, hyperesthetic	7–21 d, minimal scarring
Deep partial thickness (second degree)	Epidermis, part of dermis: epidermal-lined hair and sweat glands intact; hair follicles and glandular tissue damaged	Flash, hot liquids, hot solids, flame, and intense radiant injury	Pale/patchy cheesy white to red; wet or waxy dry, almost always blisters; no blanching	Sensitive or painful to pressure	30 d to months, late hypertrophic scarring; marked contracture formation; may require skin grafting
Full thickness (third degree)	Epidermis and all layers of the dermis; may involve subcutaneous fat, muscle, and bone	Sustained flame, electrical, chemical, and steam	Can be leathery, cracked, waxy white, cherry red, brown, or black; no blanching; no blisters	Little pain; deep pressure	Cannot self-regenerate; needs grafting; eschar can compromise viability of limb or torso if circumferential

- Any patient who sustains a severe burn (greater than 20% TBSA) is at a high risk of developing an invasive wound infection, also referred to as burn wound sepsis, which often leads to multiorgan dysfunction and death
- Early fluid resuscitation management is essential to reduce patient mortality and morbidity
- Carboxyhemoglobin saturation should be less than 10%
- Escharotomy relieves the pressure and restores perfusion to the area by releasing the constricting eschar
- Fasciotomy relieves the pressure and restores perfusion to the area but the cut is deeper than the escharotomy and goes into the muscle

REFERENCES

1. Rice PL, Orgill DP. Classification of burns. Available at: http://uptodate.com. Accessed July 18, 2012.
2. Morton P, Fontaine D. Critical care nursing: a holistic approach. 10th edition. Philadelphia: Lippincott William & Wilkins; 2009. p. 1349–73.
3. American Burn Association. Burn incidence and treatment in the United States: 2011 Fact sheet. Available at: http://www.ameriburn.org/resources_factsheet. php. Accessed September 2, 2012.
4. American Burn Association. Burn center referral criteria. Available at: http://www. ameriburn.org/BurnCenterReferralCriteria.pdf?PHPSESSID=873261082ae804192 bc5388b2899af3a. Accessed September 2, 2012.
5. Morton PG, Fontaine DK. Essentials of critical care nursing: a holistic approach. Philadelphia: Lippincott Williams & Wilkins; 2013. p. 1184–208.
6. Rice PL, Orgill DP. Emergency care of moderate and severe thermal burns in adults. Available at: http://uptodate.com. Accessed July 18, 2012.
7. Lewis, Dirksen, Heitkemper, et al. Burns. In: Lewis SL, Dirksen SR, Heitkemper MM, Bucher L, Camera IM, editors. Medical surgical nursing: assessment and management of clinical problems. St Louis (MO): Elsevier Mosby; 2011. p. 472–94.
8. Williams C. Successful assessment and management of burn injuries. Nurs Stand 2009;23(32):53–62.
9. Pham TM, Cancio LC, Gibran NS, American Burn Association. American Burn Association Practice Guidelines burn shock resuscitation. J Burn Care Res 2008;29:257–66.
10. Mandel J, Hales CA. Smoke inhalation. Available at: http://uptodate.com. Accessed July 18, 2012.
11. Peck MD. Global costs of fires and burns. Available at: http://uptodate.com. Accessed June 19, 2012.
12. Mandell SP, Klein MB. Primary operative management of hand burns. Available at: http://uptodate.com. Assessed June 19, 2012.
13. Gauglitz GG, Shahrokhi S. Clinical manifestations, diagnosis, and treatment of burn wound sepsis. Available at: http://uptodate.com. Accessed July 18, 2012.
14. Modrall JG. Lower extremity fasciotomy techniques. Available at: http://uptodate. com. Accessed July 18, 2012.

Summer Activities
Incidents and Accidents

Stephen D. Krau, PhD, RN, CNE

KEYWORDS

- Summer accidents • Drowning • Caving • Burns • Water activities • Camping
- Backpacking

KEY POINTS

- Summer is a season of unique activities and unique injuries.
- Pathophysiologic features and treatments are different for victims of freshwater and salt-water drowning.
- Treatment of drowning victims involves a comprehensive set of interventions and monitoring protocols.
- Males are more prone to water-related injuries and accidents than females.
- Drowning is a leading cause of death for children 0 to 4 years of age.
- Most burns in adults are the result of accelerant use, and usually involve alcohol.
- Children can experience severe campfire burns hours after the fire is believed to be extinguished.

INTRODUCTION

Summer encourages activities and sports that are not typically conducive to the conditions of the colder weather during other times of the year. Many of these activities involve elements of the outdoors, including water activities, hiking, biking, and camping. Also, summer is a time for outdoor cooking, campfires, and the traditional Fourth of July firework pastimes. All of these activities herald the fun of summer, but all of these have resulted in incidents and accidents. Some of these incident and accident victims present in critical care units.

DROWNING MORTALITY

According to the World Health Organization, drowning is the "process of experiencing respiratory impairment from submersion/immersion in liquid."[1] If a person dies during

School of Nursing, Vanderbilt University Medical Center, Godchaux 309, 461 21st Avenue South, Nashville, TN 37240, USA
E-mail address: steve.krau@vanderbilt.edu

Crit Care Nurs Clin N Am 25 (2013) 287–295
http://dx.doi.org/10.1016/j.ccell.2013.02.014
0899-5885/13/$ – see front matter © 2013 Elsevier Inc. All rights reserved.

the process of drowning, this is referred to as fatal drowning. If the victim is rescued, the process of drowning is interrupted and referred to as nonfatal drowning.[2] Drowning is a major global issue and it affects all age groups throughout the world, but among children younger than 15 years, there are more victims than in any other age group.[1] The World Health Organization has identified that more than 175,000 children and adolescents die each from drowning.[3,4] Drowning is the third leading cause of accidental death in the United States.[5] In the United States, the overall mortality of drowning has declined in the last decade, but remains the leading cause of accidental death among children aged 1 to 4 years.[6] During 1999 to 2006 in the United States, there were 27,514 deaths, of which 21,668 (78.8%) were males, and 4241 (15.4%) were children from 0 to 4 years of age.[4] During this period, the overall mortality has been shown to decrease by about 5%.

Although the incidence of pediatric drowning has decreased over the last decade, children younger than 4 years have the highest mortality from drowning, and are most likely to drown while bathing or from falling into water. Older children are more likely to drown in open water.[7,8] Other factors related to pediatric drowning have been identified and include lack of barriers or fencing around swimming areas, inadequate supervision, not wearing safety flotation devices, use of personal watercraft, and seizures.[9] In an estimated 30% to 50% of adolescent and adult drowning, alcohol is involved.[8]

Among males aged 5 to 19 years, the rates of mortality associated with drowning were higher among African Americans, American Indians/Alaskan Natives, and Asian/Asian Pacific Islander males than among white males. Between 2005 and 2009, the fatal drowning rate for African Americans was significantly higher than whites regardless of age. Geographically, during 1988 to 1992, the mortality related to drowning was 10 times higher in Alaska than the overall US rate.[10] Recently, the highest incidence of infant drowning in swimming pools has occurred in Florida.[4]

The Process of Drowning

The drowning process is conceptualized as a continuum that is initiated when the victim's airway is submerged in liquid, usually water.[5] Typically, the victim voluntarily holds their breath, which is followed by a laryngospasm caused by presence of liquid in the oropharynx. During the breath holding and laryngospasm, the victim is unable to breathe. This situation results in carbon dioxide accumulation and depletion of oxygen. This state results in hypercarbia, hypoxia, and acidosis.[5,11] About 10% of drownings do not involve aspiration of fluid into the lung.[12–14] This category is commonly referred to as dry drowning, which is the result of a laryngospasm from water in the upper airway and hypoxia. The remaining 90% of drownings are commonly referred to as wet drowning, in which the volume and content of the aspirated fluid cause hypoxemia.[11,15] As the victim's arterial oxygenation pressure decreases further, the laryngospasm resolves and the victim begins to inhale the liquid in which they are submerged.

Drowning events are not all the same. Depending on the type of liquid, be it seawater from the ocean, or freshwater from lakes and streams, or chlorinated water from pools, the results are different. The temperature of the water is also a determinant in the overall outcome.[5] In addition, the health of the victim, the age of the victim, and a variety of other factors make a difference in the scenario and the outcome.

Pathophysiology of Drowning

Water chemistry is a major determinant in the physiologic effects of drowning. The more rapidly freshwater enters the lungs, the more rapid the onset of ventricular fibrillation.[16] With salt water, there is diffusion, or more specifically a transudation, of fluid from the intravascular spaces into the alveoli, which results not only in pulmonary edema but also in hypovolemia.[16] If the person is rescued alive, their outcome is predominately the function of the amount of water that has been aspirated, along with its effects. Water of any sort in the alveoli results in surfactant dysfunction and washout.[2] The effects of fluid in the lungs and loss of surfactant, combined with the increased permeability of the alveolar-capillary member, result in decreased lung compliance, increased areas of low to no ventilation perfusion in the lungs, atelectasis, and bronchospasm.[17]

In rescues, the neurologic damage is similar to that of other events that warrant cardiopulmonary resuscitation (CPR). However, the temperature of the water is a factor for these victims, because hypothermia can reduce the oxygen consumption in the brain. This situation delays the cellular anoxia and depletion of adenosine triphosphate) in the brain. In a temperature-dependent fashion, hypothermia reduces the electrical and metabolic activity of the brain.[2] There is a reduction of about 5% of cerebral oxygen consumption for each 1°C in temperature that ranges from 37°C to 20°C.[18]

These factors provide the basis of much debate related to rescue attempts for submerged victims. A proposed guide for rescue suggests that when the temperature of the water is warmer than 6°C, survival or resuscitation is highly unlikely if the victim has been submerged for more than 30 minutes. If the temperature of the water is 6°C or less, survival/resuscitation is unlikely if the victim has been submerged more than 90 minutes.[19] It is evident that low ambient temperatures, low water temperatures, and perhaps, to some extent, the duration of exposure are determinants of survival. Other pathophysiologic processes are conveyed in **Table 1**.

Treatment of Near Fatal Drowning

Most episodes of drowning occur in settings that are outside a hospital, and the initial interventions for the drowned individual have a direct effect on their outcome. The goal of therapy at the initial setting is to restore ventilation and circulation, and to normalize gas exchange, as well as acid-base status.[5] CPR should be initiated immediately and can be performed in the water, if there is no danger to the rescuer. As with all persons requiring resuscitation, maintenance of an airway is essential. Current guidelines and assessment standards for CPR should be initiated as soon as possible. Unless a foreign object is obstructing the airway, the Heimlich maneuver is contraindicated.[23] Most of the water that exits the mouth during a Heimlich maneuver comes from the stomach and not the lungs, and there is a high risk for aspiration of stomach contents when the maneuver is performed.

When health care professionals and emergency equipment become available, the victim should receive 100% oxygen with a bag-valve-mask. Continuous positive airway pressure (CPAP) should be initiated. Because of the changes in intrathoracic pressures that occur during CPAP therapy, circulation parameters should be monitored. In victims who cannot protect their airway, endotracheal intubation is appropriate, with manual or mechanical ventilation as available. Although initially on intubation there may be copious amounts of pulmonary edema fluid, endotracheal suctioning can diminish the oxygenation and should be carefully considered before suctioning.[2]

If hypotension is not corrected by oxygenation, intravenous fluid therapy with normal saline should be initiated, along with inotropes, as needed.[5] Rapid fluid administration in this case should occur regardless of whether the immersion liquid is seawater or freshwater.

Table 1 Pathophysiologic effects of drowning	
Effect	**Process and Treatment**
Effects on blood-gas exchange	Hypoxia occurs immediately on aspiration of fluid. In victims who have not aspirated and are rescued in 1.5–2 min of submersion, reinstitution of ventilation and circulation immediately reverses hypoxemia.[5] When aspiration occurs, hypoxemia can persist from a few hours to weeks
Mechanism of pulmonary effects	Whether drowning occurs in freshwater or seawater, there is pulmonary edema, a decrease in pulmonary compliance, and a ventilation/perfusion mismatch. Immediately after aspiration, there is a large alveolar-oxygen gradient Pao_2 and intrapulmonary shunting can be improved by use of positive end-expiratory pressure or through the use of continuous positive airway pressure.[5] Some studies have suggested nitric oxide as a potential treatment of improving physiologic parameters, but there have not been enough rigorous studies in drowning victims to conclude the overall efficacy[20]
Changes in blood volume	If more than 11 mL/kg of hypotonic solution (freshwater) is aspirated, the blood volume increases in proportion to the amount of aspirate. When hypertonic (seawater) is aspirated, the blood volume decreases and can cause hypovolemia[16] Although most drowning victims do not aspirate quantities of fluids to cause life-threatening changes in volume, when this does occur, monitoring central venous pressure, pulmonary pressures, stroke volume variability, right ventricular end diastolic measurements, and a transesophageal echocardiography are indicated[5]
Changes in serum electrolytes	Life-threatening electrolyte changes are rarely seen in drowning victims. Electrolytes need to be evaluated Hemolysis as the result of large amount of freshwater aspiration can result in high serum potassium levels; otherwise, correction of electrolyte imbalance is rarely needed Routine use of sodium bicarbonate to correct acidosis is not commonly indicated. Correction often occurs with correction of underlying causes In cases in which intravenous fluids are indicated, the fluid should be isotonic (0.9% NaCl). Hypotonic solutions are contraindicated[5]
Effects on hemoglobin and hematocrit	In cases of large volumes of freshwater aspiration, hemolysis can occur, which increases serum hemoglobin and potassium. This situation is the result of hypotonicity and o profound hypoxemia. With severe hemolysis, profound bleeding disorders can occur
	(continued on next page)

Table 1 (continued)	
Effect	**Process and Treatment**
Effects on cardiovascular system	Large amounts of freshwater aspiration can result in ventricular fibrillation.[16] Cardiac issues can precipitate drowning events
Effects on the renal system	Renal dysfunction, although rare, may be the result of myoglobinuria caused by muscle trauma, acidosis, hypoxemia, and hemolysis[21]
Neurologic impact	Most drowning victims experience an episode of unconsciousness as the result of cerebral hypoxia.[22] There is no evidence to support the use of medications for neuroresuscitative therapy. Hyperthermia with warming, or other physiologic indigenous processes that warm the body, should be avoided

Even victims who revert to normal physiologic parameters should be taken to a tertiary-care facility. In transport, they should receive 100% oxygen, and their vital signs should be closely monitored. In many cases, there are underlying issues, even in the presence of normal physiologic parameters, that warrant evaluation in a hospital.

Hospital Care

Initial hospital treatment should focus on pulmonary support, with treatment specific to the patient's status. Laboratory values should be obtained for electrolyte and acid-base status. Continued oxygen support is indicated. All unconscious patients require intubation.[5] CPAP and positive end-expiratory pressure (PEEP) should be titrated to keep the Pa_{O_2} (partial pressure of oxygen, arterial) greater than or equal to 95%, using the lowest F_{IO_2} (fraction of inspired oxygen) setting.

In cases in which intravascular volume is an issue, hemodynamic monitoring is warranted. Although cardiac output may decrease with the introduction of CPAP and PEEP, it usually returns to normal with intravenous fluid therapy. Long-term inotropes are not usually needed.[5]

Pharmacologically, antibiotics should be initiated if the patient shows signs of infection, or if the liquid in which the drowning occurred is known to be heavily contaminated. Otherwise, antibiotic therapy should be based on the results of an obtained serum culture and sensitivity. Steroids are not usually indicated because they are ineffective in treating pulmonary lesions that occur during drowning and may inhibit the healing process. Bronchospasms, which might occur, should be treated with metered dose inhalers or nebulized albuterol.[5]

A common finding after drowning is pulmonary edema. In these cases, CPAP or PEEP facilitates oxygenation while the pulmonary tissues recover. Breaking the ventilator circuit to suction or provide nebulized treatments during CPAP and PEEP can result in recurrence of pulmonary edema and hypoxia.[5] Critical care nurses should minimize or if possible avoid any interruption of the ventilator/patient system.

There is a great deal of discussion related to placing an intracranial pressure (ICP) monitor device in drowning victims. Mild hyperventilation is known to reduce ICP in patients with cerebral edema (Pa_{CO_2} [partial pressure of carbon dioxide, arterial] at around 30 mm Hg). An ICP monitoring device should be considered if hyperventilation is considered a treatment option. As indicated by Layon and Model,[5] if ICP is increased ($\geq$20 mm Hg), the use of hyperventilation to achieve a $Paco_2$ of 25 to 30 mm Hg might decrease cerebral flow, and thus cerebral pressure, and keep the cerebral perfusion pressure (mean arterial pressure minus the ICP) at around 60 to 70 mm Hg. The use of hyperventilation to reduce ICP in drowning victims has not been proved. Mannitol should be considered if hyperventilation alone does not reduce ICP, as a bolus of 0.25 g/kg of the patient's body weight.[5] Brain damage in drowning victims is believed to be the result of hypoxia during the event, as opposed to being the result of ICP.

Prehospital care of drowning victims has a definitive impact on the overall outcome of the victim. Patients who receive effective, early basic CPR have the best chance of normal survival. Treating pulmonary and cardiovascular issues of the drowning victim in hospital is successful. The most questionable aspect related to the care and recovery of the drowning victim centers around the neurologic outcome.

CANOEING, KAYAKING, AND WHITE-WATER RAFTING INJURIES

According to the Outdoor Foundation, 23.9 million people in the United States undertake paddling activities each year. Canoeing is the most popular paddling activity (10.1 million), followed by kayaking (6.2 million).[24] The US Coast Guard in their recreational boating statistics in 2009 identified 141 deaths associated with these activities, with 89 deaths related to canoeing activities and 52 deaths associated with kayaking.[24]

There is little information about injury data related to these activities, and there is no clear distinction between these activities as recreation as opposed to sporting events. One study[25] suggests that the overall risk of injury from canoeing and kayaking is 4.5 injuries for every 1000 days of paddling. The most common injuries are the upper limb, including shoulders, wrists, hands, elbows, and forearms. Back injuries are also common and limit resuming the activity the longest.[26]

CAVING INJURIES

It is estimated that at least 2 million people in the United States visit caves each year.[27] Although the caving community does consider safety a priority, there are inherent risks involved in this summer activity. A recent study[28] indicated that most caving injuries occur during the summer months, with a peak in July. The average number of caving victims per year is 50, and the number of caving incidents is about 32 per year. Second to needing outside assistance to exit the cave (54%), the most common incident was related to caver falling, which was about 24% of the overall incidents and responsible for 74% of the traumatic injuries, with most being fractures. The most common site of these injuries was the lower extremities, followed by upper extremities and the head.[28] The incidence of fatality associated with caving is 3 deaths per year.

HIKING AND BACKPACKING

A recent study examining injuries at Yellowstone National Park that required emergency medical system activation identified that most injuries occur during the summer months.[29]

Hiking and backpacking are popular activities, and participation among Americans has increased in the last decade. It is estimated that 69.7 million people older than 16 years have hiked in the last year. With this popularity, it is important to look at the information that is available, although it is scant.

In a variety of studies, the mean age of persons experiencing injuries during hiking and backpacking is between 35.6 and 40.9 years. Most of the injuries were sustained by males (58%–64.3%).[29] Soft tissue injuries accounted for 78% of the injuries, with only 8.8% being fractures or dislocations in 1 study.[29] In another study of reported injuries, 33.75% sustained fractures, and 49.7% had a lower extremity injury.[30]

As participation in hiking and backpacking increases, it becomes more important to recognize and plan for problems associated with wilderness medicine to best ameliorate not only the incidence but also the treatment of the accidents that occur. This information can assist in hospital and prehospital service planning. The fact that most of these accidents occur during the summer is important for hospital and unit planning.

ROCK CLIMBING ACCIDENTS

Incidents related to rock climbing have been shown to occur more frequently in summer months than other times of the year.[31] Most victims related to rock climbing activities were male (78%), with most incidents occurring in the age range of 20 to 29 years (46%), followed by 10 to 19 years (21%), and 30 to 39 years (15%). Ten per cent of the incidents were among persons between 40 and 49 years of age.[31] The incidence of fatalities among all reported incidents ranges from 5.5% to 14%.[32]

BURNS

Although burns occur throughout the year, the causes of burns during the summer are primarily the result of outdoor campfires, outdoor cooking,[33] and incidents related to fireworks during holiday celebrations. In adult populations, summer burns are usually the result of the use of accelerants and often involve alcohol consumption.[34] During the summer, children are more likely to sustain burn injuries from falling into hot embers or the fire itself.[35]

Campfire injuries in adults showed increases in surface body area being burned, a higher number of procedures for treatment, longer hospitalizations, and higher complication rates when alcohol is involved.[33] This finding could be the result of the intoxicated individual having diminished judgment and sensation during the time of the injury. Persons consuming alcohol were more prone to falling into the fire, and the hands were the most commonly burned body part.[33] Many burn injuries sustained by adults are the result of use of accelerants, especially gasoline.

Children experience burns by either falling into an active fire or playing with hot coals and ashes after the fire has been extinguished. When a fire is extinguished with sand instead of water, the residual embers can cause full-thickness burns up to 8 hours later.[36,37]

In 1 study,[35] half of the children were burned by embers and ashes the morning after the campfire, when adults believed the fire had been distinguished.

SUMMARY

Summer brings a unique census population to critical care units across the United States. Because of the seasonal nature, it is helpful for the critical care nurse to have resources available to care for these unique patients. This article is not a comprehensive overview of all injuries that are sustained in summer months, but rather a view of the incidence and prevalence of some of the major injuries that occur and the patient outcomes. Having an understanding of situations that herald summer hospital admissions helps prepare the critical care nurse to care for unique incidents and accidents and to achieve the best patient outcomes.

REFERENCES

1. van Beeck EF, Branche CM, Szpilman D, et al. A new definition of drowning: towards documentation and prevention of a global health issue problem. Bull World Health Organ 2005;83(11):853–6.
2. Szpilzman D, Joost JL, Bierrens MD, et al. Current concepts: drowning. N Engl J Med 2012;366:2102–10.
3. Peden M, Oyegbite K, Ozanne-Smith J, et al. World report on child injury prevention. Geneva (Switzerland): World Health Organization; 2008.
4. Nasrullah M, Muazzin S. Drowning mortality in the United States, 1996-2006. J Community Health 2011;36:69–75.
5. Layon AJ, Modell JH. Drowning: update 2009. Anesthesiology 2009;110: 1390–401.
6. CDC. Vital signs unintentional injury deaths among persons aged 0-19 years– United States, 2000-2009. MMWR Morb Mortal Wkly Rep 2012;61:270–6.
7. Quan L, Cummings P. Characteristics of drowning by different age groups. Inj Prev 2003;9(2):163–8.
8. Bowman SM, Aitken ME, Robbins JM, et al. Trends in US pediatric drowning hospitalizations 1993-2008. Pediatrics 2012;129(2):275–81.
9. Centers for Disease Control and Prevention. Water related injuries: fact sheet. Atlanta (GA): CDC; 2009. Available at: http://www.cdc.gov/homeandrecreationalsafety/water-safety/waterinjuries-factsheet.html. Accessed February 24, 2013.
10. Lincoln JM, Perkins R, Melton F, et al. Drowning in Alaska waters. Public Health Rep 1996;11(6):531–5.
11. Modell JH, Gaub M, Moya F, et al. Physiologic effects of near-drowning with chlorinated freshwater, distilled water, and isotonic saline. Anesthesiology 1966;27: 33–41.
12. Modell JH, Graves SA, Ketover A. Clinical course of 91 consecutive near-drowning victims. Chest 1976;70:231–8.
13. Kringsholm B, Filskov A, Kock K. Autopsied cases of drowning in Denmark 1987–1989. Forensic Sci Int 1991;52:85–92.
14. Christe A, Aghayey E, Jackowski C, et al. Drowning–post mortem imaging findings by computed tomography. Eur Radiol 2008;18:283–90.
15. Modell JH, Moya F. Effects of volume of aspirated fluid during chlorinated fresh water drowning. Anesthesiology 1966;27:662–72.
16. Assolina R, Camera GL, Messina A, et al. Pathophysiology, prevention treatment of drowning syndrome. Acta Medica Mediterranea 2011;27:31.
17. Orlowski JP, Abulleil MM, Phillips JM. The hemodynamic and cardiovascular effects of near-drowning in hypotonic, isotonic, or hypertonic solutions. Ann Emerg Med 1989;18:1044–9.
18. Polderman KH. Application of therapeutic hypothermia in the ICU: opportunities and pitfalls of a promising treatment modality. Part I: indications and evidence. Intensive Care Med 2004;30:556–75.
19. Tipton MJ, Golden FS. Proposed decision-making guide for the search, rescue and resuscitation of submersion (head under) victims base on expert opinion. Resuscitation 2011;82:819–24.
20. Mizutani T, Layon AJ. Clinical applications of nitric oxide. Chest 1996;110:506–24.
21. Modell JH. The pathophysiology and treatment of drowning and near-drowning. Springfield (IL): Charles C. Thomas; 1971. p. 3–119.
22. Layon AJ, Modell JH. Drowning and near-drowning. In: Tinker J, Zapol WM, editors. Care of the critically ill patient. London: Springer-Verlag; 1992. p. 909–18.

23. Rosen P, Stoto M, Harley J. The use of the Heimlich maneuver in near drowning. Washington, DC: Institute of Medicine; 1994. p. 1–27.
24. Franklin RC, Leggat PA. The epidemiology of injury in canoeing, kayaking and rafting. Med Sport Sci 2012;58:98–111.
25. Schoen RG, Stano MJ. Year 2000 whitewater injury survey. Wilderness Environ Med 2002;13(2):119–24.
26. Kameyama O, Shibano K, Kawakita H, et al. Medical check of competitive canoeists. J Orthop Sci 1999;4(4):243–9.
27. Hooker K, Shalit M. Subterranean medicine: an inquiry into underground medical treatment protocols in cave rescue situations in national parks in the United States. Wilderness Environ Med 2000;11:17–20.
28. Stella-Watts AC, Holstege CP, Lee JK, et al. The epidemiology of caving injuries in the United States. Wilderness Environ Med 2012;23:215–22.
29. Johnson RM, Huetti B, Kocsis V, et al. Injuries sustained at Yellowstone National Park requiring emergency medical system activation. Wilderness Environ Med 2007;18:186–9.
30. Ela GK. Epidemiology of wilderness search and rescue in New Hampshire 1999-2001. Wilderness Environ Med 2004;15:11–7.
31. Lack DA, Sheets AL, Entin JM, et al. Rock climbing rescues: causes injuries and trends in Boulder County, Colorado. Wilderness Environ Med 2012;23:223–30.
32. Sedgman IB. Climbing accidents in Australia 1955-2004. Available at: http://uob-community.ballarat.edu.au/~isedgman/climbing/Accidents.pdf. Accessed February 24, 2013.
33. Nearman KC, Do VH, Olenzek EK, et al. Outdoor recreational fires: a review of 329 adult and pediatric patients. J Burn Care Res 2010;31(6):926–30.
34. Klein MB, Heimbach DM, Honari S, et al. Adult campfire burns: two avenues for prevention. J Burn Care Rehabil 2005;26:440–2.
35. Choo KJ, Fraser JF, Kimble RM. Campfire burns in children: an Australian experience. Burns 2002;28:374–8.
36. Hoang DM, Reid D, Lentz CW. Statewide ban on recreational fires resulted in a significant decrease in campfire-related summer burn center admissions. J Burn Care Res 2013;34(1):74–7.
37. Cahill TJ, Rode H, Millar AJ. Ashes to ashes: thermal contact burns in children caused by recreational fires. Burns 2008;34:1153–7.

Traumatic Brain Injury
Pathophysiology, Monitoring, and Mechanism-Based Care

Richard B. Arbour, MSN, RN, CCRN, CNRN, CCNS[a,b,*]

KEYWORDS

- Brain trauma • Primary and secondary injury • Intracranial hypertension
- Osmotherapy • Metabolic suppression • Neurological assessment
- Neurodiagnostics • Hypothermia

KEY POINTS

- Traumatic brain injury (TBI) is a significant personal and financial burden, with approximately 50,000 patients dying annually from TBI.
- Both blunt and penetrating brain trauma initiate the cascade of secondary brain injury.
- Secondary brain injury is often a process affecting relative volumes of intracranial blood, brain, and cerebrospinal fluid. Effective, mechanism-based therapies modulate relative volumes of intracranial content and control the evolution of intracranial hypertension.
- Techniques for monitoring intracranial pressure (ICP) and brain-tissue oxygen levels can yield actionable, real-time information and direct therapy. Goal-directed therapy to control ICP elevations and maintain brain-tissue oxygen levels can modulate the effect of secondary brain injury and improve outcomes.

INTRODUCTION: SCOPE OF ISSUES

Traumatic brain injury (TBI) is among the leading causes of death in patients younger than 45 years.[1] TBI is not solely a leading cause of death and disability[2] but also represents a significant financial and personal burden, both individually and on society. There are approximately 235,000 hospital admissions for patients surviving the initial traumatic event.[2] TBI has a mortality of approximately 50,000 patients; nearly 80% of patients who suffer mild to moderate TBI have neurologic sequelae 3 months after injury, many of whom require rehabilitation services.[1–3] In addition to the financial

No financial support was utilized in the authoring of this article.
The author has no actual or potential conflicts of interest with regard to the content of this article.
[a] LaSalle University, 1900 West Olney Avenue, Philadelphia, PA 19141, USA; [b] Holy Family University, 9801 Frankford Avenue, Philadelphia, PA 19114
* School of Nursing and Health Sciences, 5928 North 11th Street, Philadelphia, PA 19141, USA.
E-mail address: RichNrs@aol.com

costs of caring for the patient after TBI, there are also human costs arising from loss of employment and productivity as well as altered family dynamics, low self-esteem, and grief associated with dramatic life changes and lost potential. Severe TBI is defined as a Glasgow Coma Scale (GCS) Score of 3 to 8 out of 15.[2,4,5] Mild TBI is defined by a GCS of 13 to 15, and moderate TBI is defined by a GCS of 9 to 12.[2,4,5] A summary of the GCS is shown in **Table 1**.[2,4–6] A comparison of mild, moderate, and severe TBI is shown in **Table 2**.[2,4,5] This article reviews the pathophysiology and mechanism-based management of TBI. The scope of the discussion includes epidemiology and pathophysiology, and appropriate nursing considerations related to assessment, diagnostics, and clinical management of persons with TBI. In addition, the reader is guided through a case study to explore the application dimensions of these considerations.

TBI PATHOPHYSIOLOGY AND TRAJECTORY

TBI may be classified in two ways. In closed head injury, the brain is injured from trauma to the skull or a sudden, severe motion causing the brain to make contact by force with the inner table of the skull.[2,5,7,8] This contact may lead to direct tissue injury and capillary hemorrhage such as cerebral contusion or vascular injury, causing epidural or subdural hematoma.[5,7] A second classification is penetrating brain trauma, an injury resulting from a projectile or sharp object (generally) penetrating the scalp, cranial vault, meninges, and brain tissue itself.[9,10] This injury also exposes the intracranial cavity and its contents to the external environment.[9,10] The small cross-sectional area allows maximal delivery of force at the point of contact and maximizes penetration.[9] A Comparison of blunt versus penetrating brain trauma is illustrated in **Fig. 1**.

TBI may be further differentiated into primary and secondary brain injury.[4,5,7–9,11–13] The first stage, primary brain trauma, begins at the moment of injury and may be the result of a depressed skull fracture, closed head injury, penetrating brain trauma, subdural/epidural hematoma, and/or traumatic intracerebral hemorrhage, as well as brain contusion or laceration.[1,5,7–9,11,13] Diffuse brain injury may occur from rapid acceleration/deceleration and cause diffuse axonal injury and/or brain edema.[1,5,7,11] The second stage, secondary brain injury, begins following the immediate trauma and includes brain ischemia, autoregulatory failure, anaerobic metabolism, increased tissue lactate,[7] cellular energy failure, release of excitatory amino acids, and loss of cell membrane integrity.[8,11–13] This loss of membrane integrity allows sodium and

Table 1 Glasgow Coma Scale score		
Motor Response (M)	**Verbal Response (V)**	**Eye Opening (E)**
Follows commands: 6		
Localizing to stimulation: 5	Oriented: 5	
Withdrawal to painful stimulation: 4	Confused, appropriate: 4	Spontaneous: 4
Flexion (decorticate) posturing: 3	Disoriented, inappropriate: 3	Eye opening to voice: 3
Extensor (decerebrate) posturing: 2	Incomprehensible sounds: 2	Eye opening to stimulation: 2
No response: 1	No response: 1	No response: 1

Data from Refs.[2,4–6]

Table 2
Comparison of mild, moderate, and severe traumatic brain injury (TBI)

Index	Mild TBI	Moderate TBI	Severe TBI
Glasgow Coma Scale score	13–15	9–12	3–8
Loss of consciousness	<30 min	30 min to 24 h	>24 h
Posttraumatic amnesia	0–1 d	1–7 d	>7 d

Data from Refs.[2,4,5]

calcium influx into the cells, lipid peroxidation and, ultimately, loss of structural integrity.[1,5,7,8,11–13] Loss of structural integrity allows influx of water into the cell and subsequent progressive brain edema.[8,13] Loss of cell membrane integrity following severe TBI also activates the coagulation cascade and risks additional brain ischemia, owing to intravascular clot formation within smaller vessels.[14]

TBI affects all 3 components of the contents within the intracranial space, which include brain bulk, cerebrospinal fluid (CSF), and brain blood volume. Brain bulk (approximately 80% in stable homeostasis) increases after water influx to brain tissue and/or inflammatory response. CSF dynamics (approximately 10% in stable homeostasis) may be altered because of obstructive or communicating hydrocephalus. Brain blood volume within the arterial and venous systems (approximately 10% in stable homeostasis) may contribute to secondary injury. These conditions may be consequent to autoregulatory failure, hyperemia, and/or compromised venous drainage from the brain. Cerebral blood flow extremes of hyperemia (beyond metabolic needs) cause a risk of increase in intracranial pressure (ICP). Oligemic states of cerebral blood flow (CBF) (below metabolic needs) may result in brain ischemia. Salient events in ICP elevation and onset/progression of secondary brain injury are alterations in the relative volume of these 3 components contained within the intracranial vault.

Each component of intracranial hypertension is part of the continuum of secondary brain injury. During aggressive management of ICP elevations, multiple

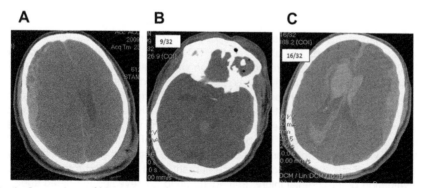

Fig. 1. Comparison of blunt versus penetrating brain trauma. (*A*) Head computed tomography (CT) of blunt brain trauma illustrating soft-tissue swelling posteriorly and significant subdural hematoma and ventricular compression of left side, with dramatic midline shift. (*B*) Head CT of penetrating brain trauma illustrating fracture of eye socket on right side with injection of bone fragments, and (*C*) consequent subdural hematoma, intraventricular hemorrhage, and midline shift. In both cases, significant sulcal effacement is evident, indicating severe brain edema/neuroimaging evidence of severe elevation of intracranial pressure (ICP).

mechanism-based interventions are used to modulate 1 or more components of intracranial pathophysiology. For example, osmotic therapy with mannitol and/or hypertonic saline creates an osmotic gradient between edematous brain tissue and circulating blood volume. This gradient facilitates water movement out of swollen brain tissue to treat brain edema. Managing increased brain blood volume includes titration of controlled ventilation and facilitation of venous drainage from the head and neck. Optimal care for intracranial hypertension and risk of herniation caused by hydrocephalus (increased relative CSF volume) includes ventricular CSF drainage managed by vigilant ICP monitoring. Metabolic suppression therapies such as barbiturates or propofol decrease the metabolic rate of brain tissue, decrease CBF, and modulate intracranial hypertension. Therapeutic hypothermia may be used for refractory intracranial hypertension to modulate the cerebral metabolic state and CBF. Aggressive normothermia protocols to protect the brain from consequences of febrile states are also used. Decompressive hemicraniectomy (increasing space available for swollen brain tissue) may be used in the management of refractory ICP elevations in select cases, pending resolution of severe brain edema.

Sedation may be part of the plan of care to decrease anxiety and brain arousal. Analgesia may be used to decrease response to noxious stimuli and blunt brain arousal. Brain arousal may increase CBF and complicate ICP control. Neuromuscular blockade may be used to eliminate patient-ventilator dyssynchrony and eliminate coughing, both of which may raise intrathoracic pressure and, consequently, ICP. Neuromuscular blockade may also be used to decrease metabolic load by paralyzing skeletal muscles. The overall plan of care for a patient following TBI is controlling the consequences of secondary brain injury, such as avoiding hypoxemia, electrolyte/acid-base imbalances, and preventing ICP progression to brain herniation syndromes. A devastating and fatal consequence of refractory ICP elevation is terminal brainstem herniation.

TBI CASE STUDY: INITIAL INJURY AND PRESENTATION

A 20-year-old white woman was transported to the emergency department (ED) by emergency medical services (EMS) in the early morning hours. She was at a social event and fell approximately 30 ft (9 m) from a balcony, sustaining closed head trauma. During transport, full cervical-spine precautions, intravenous access, and ventilation support were initiated. On arrival at the ED, airway, breathing, and circulation (ABCs) were prioritized. Controlled ventilation was initiated and maintained through an oral endotracheal tube. Early airway management and controlled ventilation is vital in avoiding hypoxemia and hypercarbia, and in modulating the progression of secondary brain injury.[15] She was initially hypotensive and tachycardic. Multiple large-bore peripheral intravenous accesses were inserted for administration of crystalloid, medications, and blood products. The patient had a GCS of 4/15, indicating severe TBI. Following volume resuscitation, her blood pressure was stabilized, ventilation was controlled, and she was transported for emergent head computed tomography (CT) for evaluation of intracranial injury. Immediate head CT revealed left-sided subdural hematoma, left frontal contusion, near total effacement of the sulci, midline shift, and compression of the ventricular system on the left side (**Fig. 2**).

The gold standard for evaluation of brain function is the clinical neurologic examination. With severe depression of consciousness, evaluation for intracranial structural lesions by obtaining emergent head CT is paramount.[16,17]

Short-term hyperventilation pending transport to the operating room (OR) for neurosurgical intervention was initiated in an effort to modulate presumed severe ICP

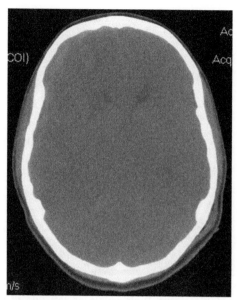

Fig. 2. Head CT obtained immediately following admission and stabilization in the emergency department. Left subdural hematoma, evolving left frontal contusion, near total effacement of the sulci, midline shift, and ventricular compression/displacement on left side.

elevations. Hyperventilation (partial CO_2 pressure [$Paco_2$] below 35 mm Hg) can result in brain ischemia, and increased morbidity and mortality. For this reason, hyperventilation is only appropriate for the shortest duration possible pending more definitive intervention for ICP elevation.[18]

Neurosurgical intervention included aggressive craniotomy without immediate replacement of the skull flap at the conclusion of surgery. This approach allowed evacuation of the subdural hematoma and insertion of a subdural drain on the operative side. **Fig. 3** illustrates immediate postoperative head CT, revealing subtotal resolution of ventricular compression/displacement and midline shift.

TBI CASE STUDY: INTENSIVE CARE UNIT MANAGEMENT IN IMMEDIATE POSTOPERATIVE PHASE

On arrival at the intensive care unit after craniotomy and drain placement, the patient received fentanyl and propofol for analgesia and sedation. This intervention was appropriate for decreasing cerebral responses to stimulation and treating pain. Neuromuscular blockade was initiated to promote synchrony with controlled ventilation, preventing surges in intrathoracic pressure consequent to cough responses and patient/ventilator dyssynchrony. Following initial operative management, clinical assessment indicated probable progression of brain edema and ICP, as evidenced by declining neurologic examination and potential brain herniation at the craniotomy site. She was transported for immediate head CT. **Fig. 4** shows the follow-up head CT, indicating an initial additional midline shift, ventricular dilatation, and brain herniation from the craniotomy defect (see **Fig. 4**A). She was immediately transported to the OR for debridement of necrotic brain tissue and ventriculostomy insertion. Postoperative head CT shows the remaining brain swelling, partial resolution of the midline shift, and placement of the ventricular catheter (see **Fig. 4**B).

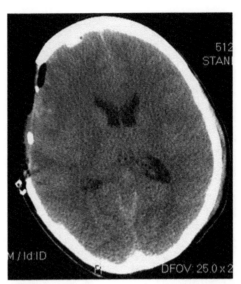

Fig. 3. Immediate postoperative head CT revealing subtotal resolution of midline shift and ventricular compression/displacement. Drain visible on left side of image in craniotomy defect.

Mannitol was titrated to a serum osmolality of 315 to 320 mOsm/L. Her controlled ventilation was titrated to maintain normocarbia ($Paco_2$ approximately 35 mm Hg). A ventilator-associated pneumonia (VAP) protocol was initiated.

Intensive Care Management

Intensive care management and postoperative care is guided as goal-directed therapy based on ICP monitoring and clinical/neurologic assessment data. ICP monitoring

A   **B**

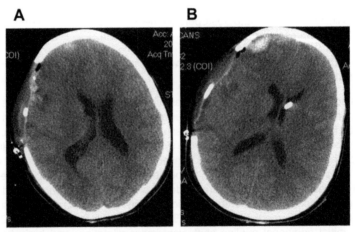

Fig. 4. Follow-up series of head CTs indicating beginning additional midline shift, ventricular dilatation, and brain herniation from craniotomy defect (*A*). Following this image acquisition, the patient was transported to the operating room for debridement of necrotic brain tissue and ventriculostomy insertion. (*B*) Postoperative head CT shows remaining brain swelling, partial resolution of midline shift and ventricular catheter placement.

may be effectively done by means of an intraventricular catheter, enabling CSF drainage and providing excellent ICP waveforms, facilitating ICP pulse-wave analysis and assessment of intracranial compliance. Other ICP monitoring options include fiberoptic catheters within the brain parenchyma. Goal-directed therapies include metabolic suppression therapies, sedation/analgesia, neuromuscular blockade (NMB), osmotic diuresis, titration of controlled ventilation, and therapeutic hypothermia in select cases.

ICP Monitoring and Waveform Analysis

Secondary brain injury may be a direct consequence of intracranial hypertension. As such, monitoring the ICP and cerebral perfusion pressure (CPP) is an immediate priority in patients following TBI.[19,20] Clinical situations whereby ICP monitoring is paramount include GCS score of 3 to 8 and abnormal head CT. ICP monitoring following TBI may be appropriate in a patient with a normal head CT if 2 of the following are present: age greater than 40 years, pathologic posturing, and/or hypotension.[19,21] ICP monitoring with frequent clinical assessment, appropriate use of imaging data, and rapid, aggressive management significantly improves outcomes.[22] Any ICP monitoring device used, to produce more benefit than harm, should be: (1) easy to use, (2) accurate, (3) interpreted within clinical context, (4) acted upon in a reproducible manner, and (5) able to guide clinical interventions.[17,23]

The most commonly used options for ICP monitoring include placement of ventriculostomy and intraparenchymal devices.[20,24] Ventriculostomy placement is considered the reference standard for ICP monitoring, giving good-quality ICP waveforms and accurate, reproducible pressure measurements.[17,19,22,24] Ventriculostomy placement allows for CSF drainage as part of mechanism-based care for the management of ICP elevations.[17,19,20,23,24] The ICP treatment threshold is generally 20 mm Hg.[17,25] ICP monitoring by means of fiberoptic intraparenchymal catheters may be initiated at the bedside and provides good-quality ICP waveforms, but does not allow CSF drainage for ICP control.[19,20,24] Placement of intraparenchymal catheters also does not require localizing the ventricular system, which may be difficult because of distortion or compression consequent to brain edema and/or space-occupying lesions.

Monitoring CPP is also integral to achieving optimal outcomes for the patient with severe TBI. CPP is determined by the following formula: CPP = mean arterial pressure (MAP) minus ICP.[17,19,22] Optimal monitoring of ICP and MAP are vital in managing severe TBI because of a twofold risk, the first of which is hyperemia consequent to hypertension and resulting surges in CBF, elevating ICP. A second risk that warrants consideration is potential for development of an oligemic CBF state consequent to systemic hypotension and resulting brain ischemia. A guideline for CPP management includes a general therapeutic range of 50 to 70 mm Hg.[26] Some clinicians advocate goal-directed therapy for CPP between 60 and 75 mm Hg.[17] In practice, CPP and ICP should be under close surveillance. As CPP trends below 60 mm Hg, identifying the cause of this clinical change and initiating appropriate intervention becomes paramount. Optimal clinical management may be directed toward ICP reduction by modulating relative volumes of CSF, brain bulk, and cerebral blood volume. Management may also be directed toward aggressive support of blood pressure by resuscitation with crystalloid/blood products or using vasoactive or inotropic agents.

In addition to ICP measurement, information may be obtained from close analysis of individual ICP pulse waveforms as well as waveform changes over time and in response to stimulation. ICP pulse amplitude reflects changes in CBF in phase with the cardiac cycle, in addition to cerebrovascular compliance and reactivity. Though requiring validation with randomized controlled study, this represents an additional approach to monitoring, yielding additional information from individual ICP pulse waveforms and concurrent MAP.[27] Additional directions for research include analysis of complexity and responsiveness of ICP trends over time and in response to stimulation, indicating probable improved states of cerebrovascular reactivity. In general, on initial study a more responsive and complex ICP is more predictive of better outcome.[28]

Close ICP waveform analysis includes evaluating individual components of the ICP pulse waveform (P-1, P-2, and P-3). P-1 reflects pulsation of the choroid plexus at cardiac systole and has the highest amplitude (under normal conditions). P-2 reflects relative brain volume and is elevated with increasing brain edema and/or rapidly expanding mass lesion. P-3 follows the dicrotic notch on the downslope of the ICP pulse waveform.[19] An elevated P-2 component of ICP pulse waveform may also indicate compromised intracranial compliance and higher predictive value for more significant ICP elevation in response to stimulation.[19] Stimulation may include airway manipulation/suctioning, repositioning, or invasive procedures such as peripheral venipuncture or thoracostomy. A comprehensive discussion of ICP monitoring is beyond the scope of this article, so the reader is referred to any of the superb reviews available.[19,20,22,23]

TBI CASE STUDY: COORDINATING ICP MONITORING WITH CSF DRAINAGE

Ventricular CSF drainage was used and guided by ICP monitoring. The ventriculostomy/transducer system was closed at intervals, and CSF was to be drained if ICP remained above 20 mm Hg for longer than 5 minutes. ICP monitoring via ventriculostomy yielded good-quality ICP waveforms, and ability to assess intracranial compliance by waveform analysis and ICP responses to stimulation with time to resolution. The patient continued to receive mannitol for hyperosmolar therapy, sedation, analgesia, and neuromuscular blockade. Protocol for prevention of VAP remained in place.

Hyperosmolar Therapy

Hyperosmolar therapy is among the mainstays of ICP control following brain trauma.[2] The 2 main options for hyperosmolar therapy are mannitol (considered first-line) and hypertonic saline.[2,4,8,10,29–33] The effect of mannitol in modulating ICP elevations is likely due to creating an osmotic gradient between circulating blood volume and an intact blood-brain barrier.[30–33] Water travels across the osmotic gradient to circulating blood volume, where it is then eliminated by the kidneys.[4,10,30–33] Mannitol provides the additional benefit of lowering blood viscosity and cerebrovascular constriction, modulating CBF and ICP.[30,31,33] Plasma volume expansion consequent to mannitol administration reduces hematocrit and blood viscosity, and increases CBF and delivery of brain oxygen.[31–33]

Close monitoring of ICP, neurologic and hemodynamic status, urine output, and serum electrolyte levels is paramount in assessing the effectiveness and duration of therapy in addition to the development of possible side effects such as electrolyte depletion, dehydration, or renal failure.[2,4,10,31,32] There is risk of rebound intracranial hypertension consequent to osmotically active molecules crossing through the blood-brain barrier leading to water influx into the brain, exacerbating brain edema and intracranial hypertension.[10,30–32] To guide therapy, serum osmolality may be raised to 320 mOsm/L.[4,30,32,33] Although typically used with and guided by ICP measurements, mannitol may be used before initiating ICP monitoring for herniation syndromes or before progressive neurologic decline is clinically evident. Mannitol dosing may be used as a low-dose (0.25 mg/kg) or high-dose (1.0 g/kg) protocol, and should be administered as an intravenous bolus 20% solution over 15 to 20 minutes.[4,30] Appropriate isotonic volume replacement and electrolyte supplementation (hypokalemia risk) are administered as appropriate.[4,32,33]

Hypertonic Saline

The effects of hypertonic saline (HTS) on modulating ICP elevations are similar to those of mannitol, mobilizing water across an intact blood-brain barrier in response to an osmotic gradient, and reducing water content in the brain.[29,31–34] Additional effects on cerebral microcirculation occur. HTS dehydrates vessel endothelium, increases plasma volume, and decreases blood viscosity, improving CBF.[31–33] HTS has been used in concentrations ranging from 1.9% to 29.2%, with variations in the total HTS volume administered.[29,30,32] HTS has been shown repeatedly to be effective in lowering ICP in patients refractory to mannitol.[30,32,34] In acute management, bolus dosing with 30 mL 23.4% saline has been effective in dramatically lowering ICP, including reversing preterminal herniation syndromes.[2,8,10,29,35] Additional clinical effects of HTS observed include significant improvements in brain oxygenation and in cerebral and systemic hemodynamics.[29,36,37] Higher concentrations may be administered through central venous access to minimize the risk of vascular injury.[2,8,30,34] Over time and with additional controlled study, including with additional patient demographics, HTS may be further validated and become first-line therapy in the aggressive management of brain edema.

Pulmonary Management and Severe Traumatic Brain Injury

Managing pulmonary physiology can be extraordinarily challenging in a patient with severe TBI. Arterial CO_2 must be closely monitored and balanced with close ventilator titration to avoid extremes of hypercapnia and hypocapnia, avoiding cerebral hyperemia versus ischemia. A second factor is clinically appropriate pulmonary care, including head-of-bed (HOB) positioning and closely following protocols to prevent VAP; this includes frequent mouth care and deep airway suctioning. Mouth care and deep airway suctioning may stimulate strong gag and cough reflexes, respectively, which may raise intrathoracic and ICPs. A third factor is ventilator management in the setting of severe respiratory failure such as acute respiratory distress syndrome (ARDS) or concurrent chest/lung trauma. Optimal ventilator management may require positive end-expiratory pressure (PEEP) and nonphysiologic ventilation modes which, with altered thoracic pressure dynamics, may complicate ICP management. Maintaining optimal oxygenation and tissue oxygen delivery is paramount in preventing secondary brain injury.

Titrating Arterial Carbon Dioxide

Hyperventilation is part of aggressive care following TBI, because with significant hypocapnia (arterial CO_2 approximately 25 mm Hg), ICP can be rapidly reduced. Hyperventilation reduces ICP because of cerebral vasoconstriction which, in a CBF state already potentially compromised, dramatically increases risk of brain ischemia.[2,10,18,38] Long-term hyperventilation is not recommended but may be appropriate in the short term to control ICP elevations, pending other mechanism-based therapeutics such as osmotherapy, sedation/analgesia, surgical intervention, or metabolic suppression therapies.[2,4,10,18,33] If available, measures to monitor brain oxygen levels may be appropriate to titrate therapy.[18,33] In general, long-term ventilation should be titrated for a $Paco_2$ of approximately 35 mm Hg, avoiding extremes of hypocapnia or hypercapnia.

Pulmonary Management over the Trajectory of Care

Integral to managing any ventilator-dependent patient are close attention to maintaining airway patency, clinically appropriate pulmonary care, and use of appropriate VAP protocols. VAP protocols include mouth care at appropriate intervals, HOB elevation of 30° or more, and prophylaxis for stress ulcers and deep vein thrombosis.[10] In the event that deep airway or pharyngeal suctioning stimulates cough or gag reflexes, respectively, sedation/analgesia and possibly NMB agents may be appropriate to control cough-induced surges in ICP and attenuate the risk of additional injury.

Ventilator Management, Respiratory Failure, and Severe TBI

Pulmonary complications may be significant in the patient following severe TBI and may be caused by pneumonia, pulmonary contusion, chest trauma, acute lung injury (ALI)/ARDS, and pulmonary edema, among others. With particular concern in ALI/ARDS, lung recruitment maneuvers, higher levels of PEEP, and nonphysiologic ventilation modes may be used to maintain oxygenation and ventilation.[39] Any alteration in thoracic pressure dynamics may be reflected in ICP elevations, and must be monitored and titrated very closely to maintain CPP.[39,40] High levels of PEEP in patients following severe TBI are not contraindicated; however, close monitoring and incremental titration are appropriate because ICP, MAP, and CPP responses are inconsistent and individualized.[40]

Sedation/Analgesia for Severe TBI

Clinically appropriate care for patients following severe TBI includes endotracheal intubation, controlled ventilation, and probable invasive procedures. Patient positioning, airway suctioning, mouth care, concurrent injury, and clinical states such as drug/alcohol intoxications versus withdrawal are all potential sources of pain and agitation.[4] Agitation and ventilator dyssynchrony can increase cerebral metabolic rate of oxygen ($CMRO_2$), ICP, blood pressure, and systemic oxygen consumption, decreasing oxygen availability to brain tissue and risking secondary brain damage.[41] Agitation is a symptom rather than a disease, and clinically appropriate care for patient agitation must differentiate and address the cause. For example, if agitation is due to alcohol withdrawal, replacement therapy with benzodiazepines may be effective. If agitation results from pain, opioid analgesia with an agent such as fentanyl is appropriate. If hypoxemia or progression of intracranial abnormality causes agitation, aggressive treatment to reverse hypoxemia and mechanism-based intervention for intracranial pathophysiology are most appropriate.[8]

Sedation/analgesia may decrease overall metabolic demand, and decrease (in a dose-related manner) $CMRO_2$, brain arousal from noxious stimulation, and patient/ventilator dyssynchrony, all of which contribute to elevated ICP.[10,32,41] Benzodiazepines such as midazolam are commonly used, short-acting agents for sedation that also provide anticonvulsant effects. Analgesia with short-acting agents such as fentanyl citrate are appropriate.[8] Fentanyl is well tolerated hemodynamically and has a shorter duration of action, facilitating neurologic assessments.[32] Propofol may be superior to midazolam in that it provides more pronounced metabolic suppressive effects and has a more predictable and shorter duration of action.[4,10,32,41] Propofol has the potential risk of propofol infusion syndrome (PRIS), reported in patients following severe TBI. PRIS is characterized by hemodynamic instability with a temporal relationship to initiation or upward titration of propofol, metabolic acidosis, hyperkalemia, rhabdomyolysis, and renal failure.[4,8,10,32,41–44] Regarding dosage, titration, and coordination of bolus versus infusion dosing of these agents for sedation/analgesia following severe TBI, there are excellent references available.[41] Paramount for clinically appropriate care is identifying the specific clinical state, using the drug class appropriately, individualizing the dosage based on patient tolerance, and exercising vigilance for possible side effects.

TBI CASE STUDY: REFRACTORY INTRACRANIAL HYPERTENSION

Over the following 2 days, ICP elevations became refractory to mannitol administration and CSF drainage. The patient was febrile to a temperature of 39.1°C and ICP elevations were 30 to 40 mm Hg with CPP 45 to 60. Multiple interventions were initiated, including metabolic suppression with sodium pentobarbital and aggressive normothermia protocol to control fever, modulating febrile-induced increases in CBF and secondary neuronal injury. To initiate drug-induced coma, the patient received pentobarbital 5 mg/kg over 30 minutes followed by an infusion of 1 to 3 mg/kg/h. The infusion was initially titrated to ICP reduction and neurologic assessment followed by bedside electroencephalography (EEG) to document the level of burst suppression. Aggressive normothermia was initiated using ice packs and a cooling blanket to reduce temperature as quickly as possible. Receiving NMB and central nervous system (CNS) depressants was effective in preventing shivering.

Metabolic Suppression Therapy Following Severe TBI

Metabolic suppression therapy is used to control refractory ICP elevations. Barbiturate therapy, in a patient-specific, dose-related manner, is used for this purpose.[4,33,41,45] Barbiturate-induced coma reduces ICP by directly modulating the brain's metabolic state, oxygen consumption, and blood flow.[2,4,8,32,33] The main side effects of barbiturate-induced coma include hypotension, which may be more pronounced in volume depletion, immune suppression, and increased risk of infection.[4,33] Hemodynamic compromise may require inotropic or vasoactive agents to maintain blood pressure.[33] Prolonged duration of action, particularly in the context of therapeutic hypothermia, may interfere with clinical neurologic evaluation and prognostication.[32] More pronounced hemodynamic instability may occur with excessive barbiturate dosing, suppressing brainstem function, vasomotor tone, heart rate, and thermoregulation.

The most commonly used agent for barbiturate-induced coma is pentobarbital sodium. Drug-induced coma is typically initiated with bolus dosing (loading dose) of pentobarbital, 5 mg/kg over 15 to 30 minutes, followed by an infusion of 1 to 3 mg/kg/h. High-dose protocol may consist of a loading dose of 10 mg/kg over 30 minutes, followed by 5 mg/kg/h infusion for 3 hours, followed by 1 mg/kg/h infusion titrated to burst suppression on EEG.[2,4,8,41,46]

Alternatively, propofol may be used for drug-induced coma. An intravenous loading dose of 2 mg/kg may be administered, followed by infusion up to 200 μg/kg/min.[2,8] In any dosing regimen for drug-induced coma, close cardiopulmonary monitoring is paramount, with high vigilance necessary in this exceedingly vulnerable population. The need for pharmacologic support of blood pressure should be anticipated, and metabolic suppression therapy should be titrated based on clinical response (ICP reduction) and diagnostic EEG or EEG-derived monitoring.[2,8,32] **Fig. 5** compares and contrasts a normal EEG trace with an EEG trace illustrating the appropriate level of burst suppression (4–6 bursts/min) during drug-induced coma for ICP control.

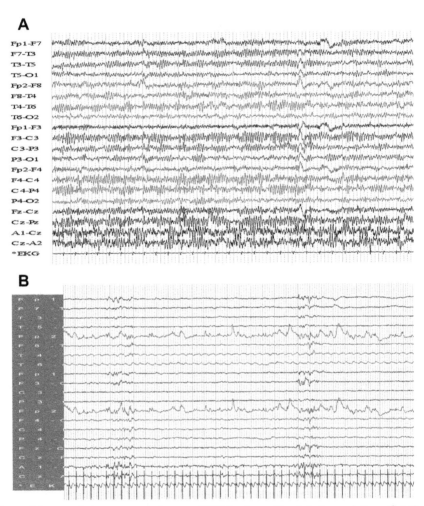

Fig. 5. (A) Normal electroencephalogram (EEG) tracing with clinical correlation of patient awake, interactive, and fully/appropriately responsive. Duration of data set 20 seconds. (B) EEG tracing illustrating appropriate level of burst suppression (4–6 bursts/min) during drug-induced coma for ICP control. EEG sensitivity on waveforms is 7 μV per millimeter.

Temperature Management Following TBI

Aggressive temperature management following severe TBI may have 2 applications, the first of which is maintaining normothermia. A second application, on a case-by-case basis, is therapeutic hypothermia. Hyperthermia or a febrile state is defined as an increase in core body temperature to more than 38.0°C. Thermoregulatory dysfunction following TBI is typically a centrally mediated phenomenon, and may result from 4 separate but related physiologic consequences: (1) direct damage to the hypothalamus, (2) excessive vasoconstriction, which limits heat loss to the environment, (3) physiologic stress mobilization and autonomic hyperactivity, and (4) an increased sweating threshold.[47] Mobilization of inflammatory response may also contribute to fever after TBI. Fever may contribute to poor outcomes by increasing neuronal hyperactivity, CBF, oxygen consumption, and ICP. It is noteworthy that brain temperature may exceed core body temperature by as much as 2°C.[48,49] Fever is strongly correlated with poor outcomes following TBI and should be aggressively treated, particularly early after injury.[48] Higher mortality, longer length of stay in hospital, and greater disability are associated with fever after TBI.[49]

Fever should be aggressively treated after TBI, because of its contribution to secondary brain injury and poor outcomes.[4,8,49] Treatment options for fever following TBI include pharmacologic and nonpharmacologic interventions. Pharmacologic interventions include acetaminophen and nonsteroidal anti-inflammatory agents.[4,8,48,49] Nonpharmacologic interventions include surface-cooling measures such as water-circulating cooling blankets, gel pads, intravascular cooling devices, and application of ice-water to skin, as well as gastric lavage and intravenous infusion with chilled fluids.[48,49]

TBI CASE STUDY: REFRACTORY INTRACRANIAL HYPERTENSION AND FEVER

Aggressive normothermia was achieved in this patient by use of a water-circulating blanket and a decrease in ambient environmental temperature, increasing the temperature gradient between the patient and environment and thus promoting heat loss. **Fig. 6** illustrates the temporal relationship between ICP reduction and the decrease in core body temperature. In the short term ICP reduction was achieved, from ICP of 35 to 40 mm Hg/T° 39.5°C to ICP of 18 to 20 mm Hg/T° 36.8°C.

Therapeutic Hypothermia

Therapeutic hypothermia (TH) is a post-TBI management option, clinically appropriate on a case-by-case basis for refractory intracranial hypertension. TH is defined as controlled temperature depression to a range between 32.0°C and 35.0°C, and routine use of prophylactic hypothermia following severe TBI is not supported by strong evidence.[50] Hypothermia use is supported in patients with significant ICP elevations refractory to other therapies such as osmotherapy, sedation/analgesia, NMB, and drug-induced coma to a state of EEG-burst suppression.[2,32] In these

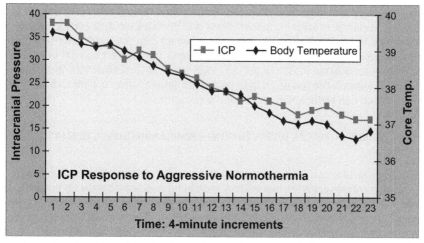

Fig. 6. Temporal relationship between ICP reduction and decrease in core body temperature.

circumstances TH has been demonstrated to reduce ICP, CBF, and mortality/severe disability 6 months after injury.[32,51] Refractory ICP elevations after TBI are associated with poor clinical and neurologic outcomes, and effective, consistent ICP control improves survival.[52]

TH produces primary neuroprotection effects by decreasing $CMRO_2$, glucose use, and lactate production. Brain oxygen consumption may decrease during TH by between 5% and 7% per 1°C decrease in temperature.[53,54] TH may also preserve high-energy phosphates, modulate gene expression, facilitate anti-inflammatory/antiapoptotic pathways, and significantly reduce ICP.[52,53,55–57] In addition, TH may stabilize the blood-brain barrier, inhibit production of free radicals, and reduce mobilization of excitatory neurotransmitters such as glutamate.[52,53,55–57]

Methods of controlled reduction of body temperature are multiple, and include internal and external cooling devices. Use of conductive techniques with devices such as cool-water–circulating blankets and gel pads applied to large skin surface areas have been used, in addition to gastric lavage with iced water, ice-water application to skin, ice-pack applications, and forced-air cooling devices.[53,54,56–58] Rapid intravenous infusion of chilled intravenous fluids such as normal saline at 3° to 4°C has been used in hypothermia initiation.[54,56,58] Intravascular devices using circulation of cold water through a catheter placed within a high-flow blood vessel such as the femoral vein have been used for rapid cooling.[54,58]

TH, though potentially helpful in managing TBI, is not a universally benign therapy. It has multiple potentially harmful side effects, and consideration of its use must be subjected to rigorous cost-benefit analysis. TH side effects include shivering (which may increase metabolic rate and interfere with TH induction), hypokalemia, decreased drug metabolism/elimination, dysrhythmias, bradycardia, decreased cardiac output/hypotension, increased systemic vascular resistance, Q-T interval prolongation, and hyperglycemia.[52,54–56,58] Coagulopathy may occur secondary to effects on platelet count, platelet function and possibly dilutional coagulopathy consequent to crystalloid administration.[52,54,58] Risk of infection such as pneumonia and wound infection is increased with TH, and increases progressively with increased duration of therapy. Gastrointestinal motility is impaired, which may have implications for initiation of feeding protocols.[52,54–56,58]

Multiple aspects of TH in the management of severe TBI remain to be refined by controlled study with larger sample sizes. Among such factors are timing and duration of therapy, optimal monitoring parameters, and therapeutic end points. Degree of temperature reduction for the optimal clinical effect may be best determined on a patient-specific basis. For example, some patients may have maximal benefit with temperature reductions to 35° to 36°C.[59] With good patient selection, available evidence does support the use of TH in patients with severe refractory intracranial hypertension, which can reduce ICP and improve outcomes.

TBI CASE STUDY: SURGICAL INTERVENTION—HEMICRANIECTOMY, HEMATOMA EVACUATION

ICP control was tenuous, as evidenced by elevated P-2 ICP waveform component and ICP elevations in response to stimulation, indicating poor intracranial compliance. On physical examination, skin overlying the craniectomy defect was tense, indicating probable high ICP and progression of brain swelling. For more definitive and long-term ICP control, additional surgical intervention was planned, including decompressive hemicraniectomy and evacuation of hematoma with possible resection of necrotic brain tissue.

Decompressive Hemicraniectomy

Intractable intracranial hypertension is one of the most dangerous secondary insults following severe TBI, and is well recognized as a significant source of mortality and morbidity.[4,32,60,61] Multiple therapeutic options are available, including surgical evacuation of intracranial lesions and modulating respective volumes of intracranial arterial and venous blood volumes, CSF, and brain tissue. In the event, intracranial hypertension remains progressive and, refractory to mechanism-based therapies, progressive injury including risk of terminal herniation syndromes can occur. One additional therapeutic option is decompressive craniectomy (DC) as rescue therapy for refractory, progressive intracranial hypertension.[57,60–62] In DC a large area of the skull is surgically removed and the dura is opened, which allows the brain to expand by increasing the relative space available to it, thus potentially controlling ICP.[4,32,57,60–62] Published studies are conflicting as regards survival and clinical outcomes in patients with TBI who were treated by craniectomy.[60–64] DC, in addition to decreasing ICP, has also resulted in sustained improvement in brain oxygenation and decreased ischemic burden.[65] Timing and patient selection are significant when determining optimal candidates for DC. Patients who still have reactive pupils and those without terminal herniation/brainstem dysfunction clearly have more chance of benefit from DC as rescue therapy.[61,66]

DC is rightly considered aggressive rescue therapy following severe TBI. It is not a benign procedure, and multiple potential complications may occur. Complications reported after DC include brain herniation through the skull defect, subdural effusion, infection, brain contusion/hemorrhage at the edge of the craniectomy defect, hydrocephalus, seizures, and ventricular enlargement.[67–69] Late complications may include cognitive dysfunction and failure of cranioplasty following skull reconstruction.[68]

TBI CASE STUDY: PRESURGICAL/POSTSURGICAL INTERVENTION

On clinical findings of compromised intracranial compliance and tense skin overlying the initial craniotomy/craniectomy defect, the patient was transported for emergent head CT. Emergent head CT (preoperative) revealed brain herniation through craniectomy defect, critical effacement of sulci, brain bleeding/contusion in the right frontal area, and near total compression of the ventricles with midline shift (**Fig. 7**A). She was transported to the OR for surgical management including resection of contused/necrotic brain areas and bifrontal decompressive hemicraniectomy. Immediate postoperative head CT revealed large frontal/temporal hemicraniectomy, partial recovery of the ventricular system, and resolution of midline shift (see **Fig. 7**B).

Following postoperative admission to the surgical intensive care unit, the patient continued to receive aggressive mechanism-based therapy for modulation of brain components including metabolic suppression. VAP protocol was maintained, as was enteral feeding. ICP was stable, and extreme vigilance was maintained for this vulnerable patient in monitoring for any possible complications.

With ICP remaining stable, intracranial compliance improving, and serial head CTs showing improving intracranial physiology, multiple steps toward recovery and ventilator liberation became possible. The first step was downward titration of neuromuscular blockade to off, with recovery of neuromuscular function as determined by clinical examination (cough, gag reflexes) initially and train-of-4 evoked responses of 4/4 at 50-mA current output. The second step was downward titration and discontinuation of pentobarbital. Clinical response was a stable ICP and marginal increase in responsiveness to stimulation with patient-triggered ventilations. The third step was

A   **B**

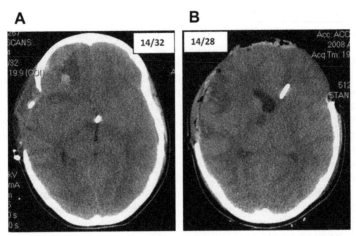

Fig. 7. (A) Emergent head CT (preoperative) revealing brain herniation through craniectomy defect, critical effacement of sulci, brain bleeding/contusion in right frontal area, and near total compression of the ventricles with midline shift. (B) Immediate postoperative head CT reveals large frontal/temporal hemicraniectomy, partial recovery of ventricular system, and resolution of midline shift.

downward titration of additional CNS depressants (fentanyl/midazolam) to off, with further increases in responsiveness.

With ICP remaining stable throughout downward titration and discontinuation of CNS depressants, and intracranial compliance recovered and stable, ventriculostomy was clamped with only intermittent monitoring. ICP was stable and lower than 20 mm Hg. Follow-up head CT revealed resolving brain edema, ventricular system symmetric and normal in size, and additional detail in sulci. Ventriculostomy was then removed, and the neurologic assessment continued to improve. Head CT after ventriculostomy removal revealed progressive resolution of brain edema and differentiation of sulci alongside a stable, symmetric ventricular system (**Fig. 8**).

The patient was increasingly responsive to family members who were in attendance in the intensive care unit throughout. It is the feeling of the author that on some level the patient had awareness of their presence during recovery, and this was one intangible factor in her favor. Ventilator weaning proceeded as clinically appropriate per protocol. Ventilator liberation was achieved, and the patient was transferred to inpatient rehabilitation. With high motivation and encouragement from her family and caregivers, and with significant hard work, she was discharged to home after inpatient rehabilitation. Ultimately she successfully returned to college.

Brain Tissue Oxygen Monitoring

All therapeutic interventions, including osmotherapy, craniectomy, metabolic suppression, and sedation/analgesia, are goal-directed approaches that aim to improve oxygen delivery and modulate the effects of ischemia at the tissue level. Mechanism-based modalities do effectively improve brain tissue oxygenation.[36,37,65,70–72]

Brain tissue oxygenation (Pbto$_2$) is measured following placement of a small oxygen-sensing probe into brain tissue. One device in common practice, the Licox monitoring system (Integra Neurosciences, Plainsboro, NJ), uses a small electrode with both temperature and oxygen sensing capability, and is placed approximately 25 to 35 mm into white matter, usually the frontal lobe.[73–76] There are multiple

A **B**

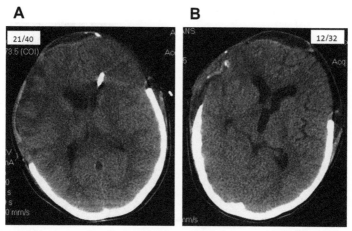

Fig. 8. (A) Follow-up head CT revealing resolving brain edema, a ventricular system symmetric and normal in size, and additional detail in sulci. (B) Head CT several days following ventriculostomy removal, revealing progressive resolution of brain edema and differentiation of sulci and a stable, symmetric ventricular system.

outstanding references with additional technical detail on the direct measurement of $Pbto_2$ including catheter placement, calibration, and imaging.[73–76] Comprehensive discussion of all these aspects is beyond the scope of this article. Clinical management of severe TBI using $Pbto_2$–directed therapy is being used increasingly. $Pbto_2$ is the product of CBF and cerebral arteriovenous oxygen difference, and is a focal measurement of tissue oxygenation. $Pbto_2$ values lower than 15 to 20 mm Hg may be considered a treatment threshold for ischemia using goal-directed therapy to increase cerebral oxygen delivery.[4,71,73,74]

Brain tissue oxygenation is responsive to global physiologic states and is influenced by other body systems. For example, systemic hypoxemia can reduce brain tissue oxygenation if oxygenation/ventilation needs are not met. Intervention to improve brain tissue oxygenation include increasing oxygen supply by titrating controlled ventilation and/or inspired oxygen; administration of packed red blood cells (PRBC) to increase oxygen-carrying capacity; metabolic suppression to decrease cerebral oxygen use; repositioning; and controlling fever. Additional interventions include hypertonic saline, augmentation of CPP, repositioning/kinetic therapy, NMB, and craniectomy.[4,37,70–74,77] A trend of $Pbto_2$, ICP, and MAP illustrating the responsiveness of $Pbto_2$ to global physiologic interventions is depicted in **Fig. 9**.

The patient in **Fig. 9** had a severe TBI consequent to a motorcycle accident (without helmet). He underwent aggressive, mechanism-based therapy for deteriorating neurologic examination post injury, including decompressive hemicraniectomy. Following Licox probe placement and initiation of $Pbto_2$-directed therapy, he recovered to reach inpatient rehabilitation.

Nursing Considerations

Care of any patient following severe TBI remains among the most challenging in critical care practice. Severe brain trauma affects all body systems and can stimulate a hypermetabolic state, complicating nutritional support. Patient risk may be due to therapeutic interventions such as airway management and invasive lines/drains, risking hospital-acquired infections such as VAP, bloodstream infections, or meningitis.

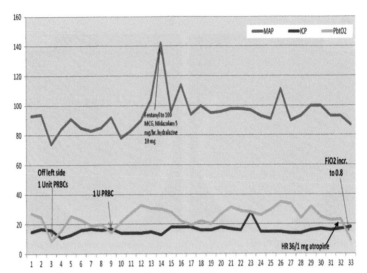

Fig. 9. Trend of brain tissue oxygenation (Pbto$_2$), ICP, and mean arterial pressure (MAP) illustrating responsiveness of Pbto$_2$ to global physiologic states and clinical interventions. PRBC, packed red blood cells; HR, heart rate.

Aggressive measures to attenuate these risks include aggressive surveillance of signs of infection, meticulous care of any invasive lines such as central venous catheters, and site rotation for peripheral intravenous catheters. Careful and frequent assessment of operative sites (craniotomy/craniectomy), ICP monitoring, and monitoring of wound and CSF drain sites are imperative. Assessment and documentation of CSF and other drainage for color, amount, character, and condition of any drain sites are vital to early identification and intervention for complications.

Surveillance of the clinical neurologic examination, trends in ICP over time and in response to stimulation, and detailed ICP waveform analysis are essential. These assessments are paramount in determining progression of injury, response to therapeutic interventions, intracranial compliance, and intracranial responses to stimulation and nursing care activities such as pulmonary care, repositioning, and tactile and auditory stimulation in a critical care area. Aggressive pulmonary care including detailed lung assessment, maintaining patient-ventilator synchrony, and monitoring oxygenation and ventilation are critical. Pulmonary physiology and intrathoracic pressure dynamics alter intracranial physiology and ICP because of risks associated with hypoxemia, hypercapnia/hypocapnia, and surges in intrathoracic pressure being transmitted to the intracranial cavity through the jugular venous system. Careful determination of actual intake/output (including potential insensible fluid losses) and judicious fluid management can maintain adequate circulating blood volume and modulate the risk of fluid/electrolyte imbalances. Aggressive feeding protocols are needed to match caloric intake with metabolic needs, particularly following severe trauma and subsequent hypermetabolic state. Early nutrition support is recommended, is associated with improved survival and decreased degree of disability, and enhances immune function.[32] Maintaining close control of blood glucose levels by titrating insulin therapy is also appropriate.[32] Hyperglycemia is associated with progression of secondary brain injury and worse outcomes.[32,78] Deep vein thrombosis prophylaxis is appropriate. Nonpharmacologic interventions such as sequential compression devices and pharmacologic interventions such as unfractionated heparin or low molecular weight heparin are options.[8,32,78] Seizure risk may be reduced after TBI by administration of anticonvulsant agents such as levetiracetam, carbamazepine, or valproic acid, as clinically appropriate, owing to the risk of secondary brain damage.[8,79]

Nursing Considerations and Family Needs

Nursing considerations are not limited to aggressive monitoring, medication administration, and management of complications. The patient's experience of severe TBI produces a cascade of effects within the family system. The family may experience almost unendurable stress, anticipatory grief, and significant fear seeing someone they love so critically ill and vulnerable. Providing spiritual support (chaplaincy) services may comfort family members and help establish rapport between the family and members of the health care team. Providing regular updates at an appropriate level of understanding may help establish and maintain trust and, possibly, decrease anxiety. It is reported that families consistently need information and professional support from the team, desire at least some involvement in care, and experience significant uncertainty during a family member's critical illness.[80] Nursing implications for families include careful education, expression of caring behaviors, involving families in care as appropriate, being aware of one's own anxiety and how it may affect families, and maintaining open communication while not avoiding families.[81]

SUMMARY

Patients in the aftermath of severe TBI are among the most challenging and vulnerable populations in critical care practice. Primary brain injury typically begins the cycle of secondary brain injury which, if progressive and refractory to therapy, can prove fatal. Secondary brain injury may arise from evolving intracranial pathophysiology and from other body systems including pulmonary, cardiovascular, neuroendocrine, and gastrointestinal dysfunction, as well as hospital-acquired infections. For these reasons, optimal care of the patient following severe TBI must include aggressive, mechanism-based therapeutics for intracranial pathophysiology, aggressive surveillance of neurologic assessment data, and meticulous assessment and care of all body systems. Multidisciplinary collaboration and effective communication are key to rapid recognition of clinical changes quickly coupled with optimal clinical management in pursuit of neurologic recovery. Family needs are also key to long-term recovery. Family communication and involvement in care are clinically appropriate, and updates help to significantly build trust, which can only help with family interaction during a critical illness.

REFERENCES

1. Pangilinan PH. Classification and complications of traumatic brain injury. Emedicine.medscape.com. Available at: http://emedicine.medscape.com/article/326643-overview#aw2aab6b2. Accessed May 1, 2012.
2. DeCuypere M, Klimo P. Spectrum of traumatic brain injury from mild to severe. Surg Clin North Am 2012;92(4):939–57.
3. Badgiata N, Carney N, Crocco TJ, et al. Guidelines for prehospital management of traumatic brain injury; 2nd edition. Prehosp Emerg Care 2007;12(Suppl 1): S1–52.

4. Haddad SH, Arabi YM. Critical care management of severe traumatic brain injury in adults. Scand J Trauma Resusc Emerg Med 2012;20(12):12. http://dx.doi.org/10.1186/1757-7241-20-12.

5. Dawodu ST. Traumatic brain injury (TBI)—definition, epidemiology, pathophysiology. Emedicine.medscape.com. Available at: http://emedicine.medscape.com/article/326510-overview#aw2aab6b3. Accessed May 1, 2012.

6. Teasdale G, Jennett B. Assessment of coma and impaired consciousness. Lancet 1974;2(7282):81–4.

7. Rangel-Castilla L. Closed head trauma. Emedicine.medscape.com. Available at: http://emedicine.medscape.com/article/251834-overview#a0104. Accessed May 2, 2012.

8. Ling GS, Marshall SA. Management of traumatic brain injury in the intensive care unit. Neurol Clin 2008;26(2):409–26.

9. Santiago LA, Oh BC, Dash PK, et al. A clinical comparison of penetrating and blunt traumatic brain injuries. Brain Inj 2012;26(2):107–25.

10. Griffin LJ, Hickey JV. Penetrating head injury. Crit Care Nurs Q 2012;35(2): 144–50.

11. Werner C, Engelhard K. Pathophysiology of traumatic brain injury. Br J Anaesth 2007;99:4–9.

12. Sahuquillo J, Vilalta A. Cooling the injured brain: how does moderate hypothermia influence the pathophysiology of traumatic brain injury? Curr Pharm Des 2007;13(22):2310–22.

13. Greve MW, Zink BJ. Pathophysiology of traumatic brain injury. Mt Sinai J Med 2009;76:97–104.

14. Chodobski A, Zink BJ, Szmydynger-Chodobska J. Blood-brain barrier pathophysiology in traumatic brain injury. Transl Stroke Res 2011;2(4):492–516.

15. Harris T, Davenport R, Hurst T, et al. Improving outcome in severe trauma: trauma systems and initial management-intubation, ventilation an resuscitation. Postgrad Med J 2012;88:588–94.

16. Tsang KK, Whitfield PC. Traumatic brain injury: review of current management strategies. Br J Oral Maxillofac Surg 2012;50:298–308.

17. Schimpf MM. Diagnosing increased intracranial pressure. J Trauma Nurs 2012; 19(3):160–7.

18. Brain Trauma Foundation. Guidelines for the management of severe traumatic brain injury, 3rd edition. Hyperventilation. J Neurotrauma 2007;24(Suppl 1):S87–90.

19. Arbour R. Intracranial hypertension: monitoring and nursing assessment. Crit Care Nurse 2004;24(5):19–32.

20. Vender J, Waller J, Dhandapani K, et al. An evaluation and comparison of intraventricular, intraparenchymal and fluid-coupled techniques for intracranial pressure monitoring in patients with severe traumatic brain injury. J Clin Monit Comput 2011;25:231–6.

21. Brain Trauma Foundation. Guidelines for the management of severe traumatic brain injury, 3rd edition. Indications for intracranial pressure monitoring. J Neurotrauma 2007;24(Suppl 1):S37–44.

22. Feyen BF, Sener S, Jorens PG, et al. Neuromonitoring in traumatic brain injury. Minerva Anestesiol 2012;78(8):949–58.

23. Mendolson AA, Gillis C, Henderson WR, et al. Intracranial pressure monitors in traumatic brain injury: a systematic review. Can J Neurol Sci 2012;39(5):571–6.

24. Brain Trauma Foundation. Guidelines for the management of severe traumatic brain injury, 3rd edition. Intracranial pressure monitoring technology. J Neurotrauma 2007;24(Suppl 1):S45–54.

25. Brain Trauma Foundation. Guidelines for the management of severe traumatic brain injury, 3rd edition. Intracranial pressure thresholds. J Neurotrauma 2007; 24(Suppl 1):S55–8.
26. Brain Trauma Foundation. Guidelines for the management of severe traumatic brain injury, 3rd edition. Cerebral perfusion thresholds. J Neurotrauma 2007; 24(Suppl 1):S59–64.
27. Aries MJ, Czosnyka M, Budohoski KP, et al. Continuous monitoring of cerebro-vascular reactivity using pulse waveform of intracranial pressure. Neurocrit Care 2012;17(1):67–76.
28. Lu CW, Czosnyka M, Shieh JS, et al. Complexity of intracranial pressure corre-lates with outcome after traumatic brain injury. Brain 2012;135:2399–408.
29. Protheroe RT, Gwinnutt CL. Early hospital care of severe traumatic brain injury. Anaesthesia 2011;66:1035–47.
30. Ropper AJ. Hyperosmolar therapy for raised intracranial pressure. N Engl J Med 2012;367(8):746–52.
31. Brain Trauma Foundation. Guidelines for the management of severe traumatic brain injury, 3rd edition. Hyperosmolar therapy. J Neurotrauma 2007;24(Suppl 1):S14–20.
32. Helmy A, Vizcaychipi M, Gupta AK. Traumatic brain injury: intensive care man-agement. Br J Anaesth 2007;99(1):32–42.
33. Honeybul S. An update on the management of traumatic brain injury. J Neurol Sci 2011;55(4):343–55.
34. Sakellaridis N, Pavlou E, Karatzas S, et al. Comparison of mannitol and hyper-tonic saline in the treatment of severe brain injuries. J Neurosurg 2011;114(2): 545–8.
35. Kerwin AJ, Schinco MA, Tepas JJ. The use of 23.4% hypertonic saline for the management of elevated intracranial pressure in patients with severe traumatic brain injury: a pilot study. J Trauma 2009;67(2):277–82.
36. Oddo M, Levine JM, Frangos S, et al. Effect of mannitol and hypertonic saline on cerebral oxygenation in patients with severe traumatic brain injury and re-fractory intracranial hypertension. J Neurol Neurosurg Psychiatry 2009;80(8): 916–20.
37. Rockswold GL, Solid CA, Parades-Andrade E, et al. Hypertonic saline and its effect on intracranial pressure, cerebral perfusion and brain tissue oxygen. Neurosurgery 2009;65(6):1035–41.
38. Rangel-Castilla L, Lara LR, Gopinath S, et al. Cerebral hemodynamic effects of acute hyperoxia and hyperventilation after severe traumatic brain injury. J Neurotrauma 2010;27:1858–63.
39. Lee K, Rincon F. Pulmonary complications in patients with severe brain injury. Crit Care Res Pract 2012;2012. http://dx.doi.org/10.1155/2012/207247.
40. Zhang XY, Yang ZJ, Wang QX, et al. Impact of positive end-expiratory pressure on cerebral injury patients with hypoxemia. Am J Emerg Med 2011;29:699–703.
41. Brain Trauma Foundation. Guidelines for the management of severe traumatic brain injury, 3rd edition. Anesthetics, analgesics and sedatives. J Neurotrauma 2007;24(Suppl 1):S71–6.
42. Diedrich DA, Brown DR. Analytic reviews: propofol infusion syndrome in the ICU. J Intensive Care Med 2011;26(2):59–72.
43. Ilyas MIM, Balacumaraswami L, Palin C, et al. Propofol infusion syndrome in adult cardiac surgery. Ann Thorac Surg 2009;87:1–3.
44. Zaccheo MM, Bucher DH. Propofol infusion syndrome: a rare complication with potentially fatal results. Crit Care Nurse 2008;28(3):18–25.

45. Stocchetti N, Zanaboni C, Colombo A, et al. Refractory intracranial hypertension and "second-tier" therapies in traumatic brain injury. Intensive Care Med 2008; 34:461–7.

46. Marshall GT, James RF, Landman MP, et al. Pentobarb coma for refractory intracranial hypertension after severe traumatic brain injury: mortality predictions and one-year outcomes in 55 patients. J Trauma 2010;69(2):275–83.

47. Sessler DI. Thermoregulatory defense mechanism. Crit Care Med 2009; 37(Suppl 7):S203–10.

48. Badjatia N. Hyperthermia and fever control in brain injury. Crit Care Med 2009; 37(Suppl 7):S250–7.

49. Mcilvoy L. Fever management in patients with brain injury. AACN Adv Crit Care 2012;23(2):204–11.

50. Brain Trauma Foundation. Guidelines for the management of severe traumatic brain injury, 3rd edition. Prophylactic hypothermia. J Neurotrauma 2007; 24(Suppl 1):S21–5.

51. Kramer C, Freeman WD, Larson JS, et al. Therapeutic hypothermia for severe traumatic brain injury: a critically appraised topic. Neurologist 2012;18(3): 173–7.

52. Sadaka F, Veremakis C. Therapeutic hypothermia for the management of intracranial hypertension in severe traumatic brain injury: a systematic review. Brain Inj 2012;26(7–8):899–908.

53. Faridar A, Bershad EM, Emiru T, et al. Therapeutic hypothermia in stroke and traumatic brain injury. Front Neurol 2011;2(Art 80):1–11.

54. Varon J, Acosta P. Therapeutic hypothermia: past, present and future. Chest 2008;133(5):1267–74.

55. Rupich K. The use of hypothermia as a treatment for traumatic brain injury. J Neurosci Nurs 2009;41(3):159–67.

56. Jiang J. Clinical study of mild hypothermia treatment for severe traumatic brain injury. J Neurotrauma 2009;26:399–406.

57. Meyer MJ, Megyesi J, Meythaler J, et al. Acute management of acquired brain injury part I: an evidence-based review of non-pharmacological interventions. Brain Inj 2010;24(5):694–705.

58. Polderman KH, Herold I. Therapeutic hypothermia and controlled normothermia in the intensive care unit: practical considerations, side effects and cooling methods. Crit Care Med 2009;37(3):1101–20.

59. Tokutomi T, Miyagi T, Takeuchi Y, et al. Effect of 35°C hypothermia on intracranial pressure and clinical outcome in patients with severe traumatic brain injury. J Trauma 2009;66(1):166–73.

60. Cianci G, Bonizzoli M, Zagli G, et al. Late decompressive craniectomy after traumatic brain injury: neurological outcome at 6-months after ICU discharge. J Trauma Manag Outcomes 2012;6:8. Available at: http://www.trauma management.org/content/6/1/8. Accessed December 22, 2012.

61. Bao Y, Liang Y, Gao G, et al. Bilateral decompressive craniectomy for patients with malignant diffuse brain swelling after severe traumatic brain injury: a 37-case study. J Neurotrauma 2010;27:341–7.

62. Olivecrona M, Rodling-Wahlstrom M, Naredi S, et al. Effective ICP reduction by decompressive craniectomy in patients with severe traumatic brain injury treated by and ICP-targeted therapy. J Neurotrauma 2007;24(6): 927–35.

63. Cooper DJ, Rosenfeld JV, Murray L, et al. Decompressive craniectomy in diffuse traumatic brain injury. N Engl J Med 2011;364(16):1493–502.

64. Eberle BM, Schnuriger B, Inaba K, et al. Decompressive craniectomy: surgical control of traumatic intracranial hypertension may improve outcome. Injury 2010;41:894–8.

65. Weiner GM, Lacey MR, Mackenzie L, et al. Decompressive craniectomy for elevated intracranial pressure and its effect on the cumulative ischemic burden and therapeutic intensity levels after severe traumatic brain injury. Neurosurgery 2010;66(6):1111–9.

66. Yatsusige H, Takasato H, Hayakawa T, et al. Prognosis for severe traumatic brain injury patients treated with bilateral decompressive craniectomy. Acta Neurochir Suppl 2010;106:265–70.

67. Honeybul S, Ho KM. Long-term complications of decompressive craniectomy for head injury. J Neurotrauma 2011;28:929–35.

68. Silver SI. Complications of decompressive craniectomy for traumatic brain injury. Neurosurg Focus 2009;26:1–16.

69. Honeybul S. Complications of decompressive craniectomy for head injury. J Clin Neurosci 2010;17:430–5.

70. Pascual JL, Georgoff P, Maloney-Wilensky E, et al. Reduced brain tissue oxygen in traumatic brain injury: are most commonly used interventions successful? J Trauma 2011;70(3):535–46.

71. Spiotta AM, Stiefel MF, Gracias VH, et al. Brain tissue oxygen-directed management and outcome in patients with severe traumatic brain injury. J Neurosurg 2010;113(3):571–80.

72. Chen HI, Malhotra NR, Oddo M, et al. Barbiturate infusion for intractable intracranial hypertension and its effect on brain oxygenation. Neurosurgery 2008; 63(5):880–7.

73. Bader MK. Recognizing and treating ischemic insults to the brain: the role of brain tissue oxygen monitoring. Crit Care Nurs Clin North Am 2006;18:243–56.

74. Littlejohns LR, Bader MK, March K. Brain tissue oxygen monitoring in severe brain injury, I: research and usefulness in critical care. Crit Care Nurse 2003; 23(4):17–25.

75. Stewart C, Haitsma L, Zador Z, et al. The new Licox combined brain tissue oxygen and brain temperature monitor: assessment of in vitro accuracy and clinical experience in severe traumatic brain injury. Neurosurgery 2008;63(6): 1159–64.

76. Barazangi N, Hemphill JC. Advanced cerebral monitoring in neurocritical care. Neurol India 2008;56(4):405–14.

77. Bader MK, Littlejohns LR, March K. Brain tissue monitoring in severe brain injury II: implications for critical care teams and case study. Crit Care Nurse 2003; 23(4):29–44.

78. Brain Trauma Foundation. Guidelines for the management of severe traumatic brain injury, 3rd edition. Nutrition. J Neurotrauma 2007;24(Suppl 1):S77–82.

79. Brain Trauma Foundation. Guidelines for the management of severe traumatic brain injury, 3rd edition. Antiseizure prophylaxis. J Neurotrauma 2007;24 (Suppl 1):S83–6.

80. Keenan A, Joseph L. The needs of family members of severe traumatic brain injury during critical and acute care: a qualitative study. Can J Neurosci Nurs 2010;32(3):25–35.

81. Yetman L. Caring for families: double binds in neuroscience nursing. Can J Neurosci Nurs 2009;31(1):22–9.

Fracture Complications

Kristen Hershey, MSN, RN

KEYWORDS

- Fracture complications • Acute compartment syndrome • Fat embolism syndrome

KEY POINTS

- This article highlights 2 important complications of fracture: acute compartment syndrome and fat embolism syndrome (FES).
- FES is most commonly associated with long-bone and pelvic fracture, whereas acute compartment syndrome is often associated with tibia or forearm fracture.
- The onset of both of these complications may be difficult to assess in the nonverbal patient or in the patient with multiple trauma.
- Careful, serial assessment of the patient with fracture is necessary to recognize and treat these complications promptly.
- Early treatment and supportive care are crucial to positive outcomes for patients with complications of fracture.

INTRODUCTION

Summer is a time for outdoor activities, recreation, sports, and travel; however, it is also a time for increased incidence of injury. Unintentional injury has significant effects to health. It is the leading cause of death for people ages 1 to 44[1] and the fifth leading cause of death for all ages.[1] In addition approximately 11,000 people seek treatment in emergency departments (EDs) daily in the United States for sports, recreation, and exercise-related injuries.[2] Unintentional injury includes accidents, such as motor vehicle collisions (MVCs), falls, and crush injuries. Although all body systems can be affected by unintentional injury, the musculoskeletal system is often impacted. One commonly encountered accidental injury to the musculoskeletal system is fracture. Complications of fracture, such as acute compartment syndrome and fat embolism syndrome (FES), require prompt recognition and intervention to prevent further injury to the patient. This article describes the pathophysiology, clinical and diagnostic findings, and treatment associated with these complications of fracture.

TYPES OF FRACTURE

Fracture to a healthy bone, as opposed to fracture of diseased bone (pathologic fracture), is classified as a "common fracture."[3] Although a full discussion of fracture is

Austin Peay State University, School of Nursing, 982 Haggard Drive, PO Box 4658, Clarksville, TN 37044, USA
E-mail address: hersheyk@apsu.edu

Crit Care Nurs Clin N Am 25 (2013) 321–331
http://dx.doi.org/10.1016/j.ccell.2013.02.004
0899-5885/13/$ – see front matter © 2013 Elsevier Inc. All rights reserved.

outside the scope of this article, it is helpful to recognize the major characteristics of various types of fractures. Descriptors of fracture type can alert the nurse to the severity of the injury, possible associated trauma, and common complications. Fracture is described by the name of the involved bone, the location of the fracture on the bone, the orientation of the fracture line, and the condition of the tissue overlying the bone.[3,4] Examples of the information that can be obtained from descriptions of fracture include the following:

- Location: The bone involved in the fracture can alert the practitioner to the presence of associated injuries. For example, pelvic fracture may have associated abdominal injuries and risk of hemorrhage, whereas tibia fractures are at high risk of compartment syndrome and osteomyelitis.[3,5] Femur and pelvic fractures have a higher risk of FES.[6]
- Orientation of fracture line: Fractures can be described as transverse, oblique, or spiral. Oblique and spiral fractures indicate a significant amount of force and associated soft tissue injury. In addition, fractures that cause displacement of the bone, or that create fragments of bone (comminuted or segmental fractures) are also associated with increased force and underlying soft tissue injury.[4]
- Skin integrity: An open fracture includes any fracture in which the skin is disrupted. Often the disruption is not dramatic and appears only as a puncture or laceration.[4] An open fracture indicates a high risk for osteomyelitis, compartment syndrome, and neurovascular damage.[4,7] A closed fracture carries an increased risk for FES.

COMPLICATIONS OF FRACTURE

Fracture may be an acute life-threatening event if it affects airway or breathing, or if it involves significant blood loss. All trauma patients should be assessed using a systematic approach, such as the ABCDE method, evaluating airway, breathing, circulation, disability, and exposure/environmental control.[8] Fracture may also result in less immediate complications that may cause significant morbidity and mortality. Two severe complications of fracture are compartment syndrome and FES. These complications can result in loss of limb function, or even death, if unrecognized or untreated. Recognition of fracture complications requires careful nursing assessment and prompt intervention to reduce the risk of morbidity and mortality for the patient.

PATHOPHYSIOLOGY OF ACUTE COMPARTMENT SYNDROME

German physician Richard Von Volkmann first described compartment syndrome in 1881.[7] He noted that what is now called Volkmann ischemic contracture was a result of an interruption of the blood supply to the forearm.[5] It is currently recognized that acute compartment syndrome most commonly results from traumatic injury to the lower leg at the tibia,[9] followed by injury to the forearm.[5]

The lower leg contains 4 compartments: the anterior, lateral, superficial posterior, and deep posterior.[7] The forearm includes 3 compartments: the flexor, extensor, and mobile wad. These compartments are composed of muscles, nerves, blood vessels, and bone, and are surrounded by relatively inelastic fascia.[10] Compartment syndrome results when the tissue pressure in one of the compartments exceeds the perfusion pressure.[9] Pressure in the compartment can be increased by internal forces, such as bleeding or edema, or may be the result of external forces, such as a tight cast or dressing.[7,11] The lower leg and forearm are more at risk for elevated pressures than other muscle compartments, such as the upper leg, because of their smaller size.[7]

Patients with larger muscle mass, particularly men younger than 35, are also at increased risk of compartment syndrome.[11]

The pathophysiology of compartment syndrome is not completely understood[5,11]; however, the arteriovenous gradient theory appears to play a key role in the development of compartment syndrome.[5,11] Increased tissue pressure leads to increased venous pressure within the compartment. As the venous pressure reaches that of the arterial pressure, the blood supply to the compartment decreases.[5] Ischemia causes lysis of the myocytes, as well as increased capillary permeability, resulting in worsening pressure and further decreasing the arteriovenous gradient.[5,11] The increased metabolic demands of the damaged tissue may also contribute to the ischemic process.[11]

Normal compartment pressure is lower than 10 mm Hg, but pressures of up to 20 mm Hg are generally tolerated without ischemia or muscle damage.[7] Because of the role of the arteriovenous gradient, however, it is currently understood that the difference between diastolic blood pressure and compartment pressure (delta pressure) is a better measure of compartment syndrome risk than compartment pressure alone.[7,11] Points to consider regarding delta pressure include the following:

- Delta pressure = diastolic blood pressure – compartment pressure.[11]
- Lower delta pressures (<30 mm Hg) have increased risk for compartment syndrome.[7,11]
- Hypotensive patients cannot tolerate increases to compartment pressure as well as normotensive patients, and are at increased risk for compartment syndrome.[5,7]

CLINICAL FINDINGS OF ACUTE COMPARTMENT SYNDROME

Acute compartment syndrome is most common in patients with significant trauma.[11] Fracture is present in approximately 75% of cases of acute compartment syndrome,[11] most commonly fractures of the tibia, followed by fractures of the forearm.[5,9,11] However, the presence of crush injuries (with or without fracture), burns, penetrating trauma, vascular injury, snake bites, or extravasation of intravenous fluids or medications may also result in acute compartment syndrome.[10,11] The "P"s of compartment syndrome are often used to direct the clinician to assessment findings indicating compartment syndrome. These often include: pain, pallor, pulselessness, paresthesia, paralysis, and poikilothermia. Other sources include palpation as an additional piece of assessment data. However, these findings do not have equal weight in recognizing acute compartment syndrome. Some are late findings, after ischemia and necrosis have occurred. Others are not found consistently, even in advanced stages of compartment syndrome.[11] Although measurement of compartment pressure is the only way to definitively establish a diagnosis,[11,12] evaluation of the "P"s of compartment syndrome is still an important bedside tool, as it may identify a need for more invasive measurement of compartment pressure.

Pain is an important, early finding in compartment syndrome.[7,11,13] The pain of acute compartment syndrome is often described as "out of proportion to the injury" and is typically unrelieved, even by narcotic pain medication.[7,12] The pain of neurovascular impairment is mediated by A-delta fibers, which do not have opioid receptors.[12] Therefore, pain is not relieved with analgesia. Acute compartment syndrome pain is increased with passive motion.[7,11,12] Pain may be masked because of the effects of sedation or decreased level of consciousness in the critical care patient.[11,12] Pain may also be difficult to assess in the patient with multiple trauma, in young children, or in other nonverbal patients.[11,12] Pain associated with acute compartment syndrome typically occurs within hours of injury, but may develop up to 48 hours after injury.[7,11] Whenever possible, pain should be evaluated consistently by self-report of pain using a validated pain assessment scale.[12] Evaluation of pain in the sedated or nonverbal patient requires alternative assessments, such as validated critical-care pain assessment tools[14] or by nonverbal signs such as grimacing, guarding, restlessness (Johnson-walker), muscle tension, and ventilator compliance.[14] Physiologic symptoms of pain, such as tachycardia, tachypnea, hypertension, and diaphoresis, should also be noted, although these symptoms are not specific only to pain.[12]

Parasthesia or paralysis are both indicative of diminished function of nerves, which are very sensitive to changes in compartment pressure.[12] The presence of parasthesia, including numbness, tingling, or decreased sensation, should be assessed frequently in the patient at risk for compartment syndrome. The presence of parasthesia is an early finding in compartment syndrome,[12] typically occurring 30 minutes to 2 hours of rising compartment pressure.[11] Knowledge of the sensory nerves most commonly affected can assist in focusing the assessment. In a patient with a lower extremity fracture, the deep peroneal and tibial nerve function may be compromised.[9] In the responsive patient, sensation should be assessed between the first and second toe, for the deep peroneal nerve, and on the sole of the foot, for the tibial nerve.[9] Paralysis is a later sign of nerve or muscle damage in compartment syndrome.[12] In the patient with lower extremity injury, this can be assessed by flexion and extension of the foot.

In the patient with forearm injury, function of the radial, median, and ulnar nerves should be assessed. In the alert patient, this can be accomplished by testing sensation between the thumb and index finger (radial), the tip of the index finger (median), and the tip of the little finger (ulnar).[7] Motor function can be assessed by asking the patient to extend the wrist and fingers against resistance, to touch the thumb and index finger together (making the "OK" sign), and to abduct the index finger against resistance.[7]

Pallor, pulselessness, and poikilothermia are late findings indicating decreased tissue perfusion and possibly irreversible damage.[10,13] A cool, pale extremity should be evaluated for surgical intervention immediately. Pulses distal to the injury should be evaluated frequently. The strength of pulses, including any changes or use of a Doppler, should be noted.[9] As always, the affected limb should be compared with the other extremity to help differentiate pathologic changes from a normal physiologic response (to a cool environment, for example).

Palpation is a tool that may be used at the bedside; however, studies have shown that palpation may not be sensitive or specific enough to reliably diagnose compartment syndrome.[11] The presence of tenseness, firmness, or a "woodenlike" feel to the extremity should alert the provider to the need for more invasive assessment.[11] These assessment findings may be particularly useful in the nonverbal or sedated patient, in whom pain and paresthesia are more difficult to identify. In the alert, verbal patient, tenderness with palpation is a common finding.[7]

Assessment findings associated with compartment syndrome are highlighted in **Table 1**.

LABORATORY AND DIAGNOSTIC TESTING FOR COMPARTMENT SYNDROME

Measurement of compartment pressure is the most reliable and sensitive method to diagnose compartment syndrome.[11] Methods of measurement include commercial handheld manometer devices, a simple needle manometer system, and a slit catheter technique. All 3 types of measurement are low-risk procedures that appear to have equal reliability.[11] If handheld manometer devices are not readily available at a facility,

Table 1
Compartment syndrome assessment findings

	Assessment Findings	Nursing Considerations
Earlier findings	Pain	Common, early finding. Out of proportion to injury, unrelieved by narcotics. May be masked by multiple trauma, sedation, or decreased level of consciousness. Increased with passive range of motion.
	Paresthesia	Early finding. Assess for decreased sensation, decreased 2-point discrimination, and "pins and needles."
	Palpation	Unreliable sensitivity and specificity, but may be used to assess for changes. Firmness, woodenness, and pain with palpation may indicate rising compartment pressure.
Later findings	Paralysis	Later sign indicating possibly irreversible nerve or muscle damage.
	Pallor	Later sign indicating poor perfusion. Assess in relation to opposite extremity.
	Pulselessness	Later sign indicating poor perfusion. Assess serially and note changes to strength or use of Doppler device.
	Poikilothermia	Later sign indicating poor perfusion. Assess in relation to opposite extremity. Consider environmental causes.

the simple needle system has the advantage of using equipment readily available in the critical care setting. In this procedure, the clinician measures compartment pressure using an 18-gauge needle attached to an arterial pressure monitor.[11] Normal tissue pressure ranges from 0 to 8 mm Hg.[11] Multiple pressure measurements may be required and pressure should always be considered in light of other clinical findings.[7,11] Measurement should be obtained within 5 cm of the fracture site.[7] Measurement farther from the fracture site decreases accuracy.[11]

Laboratory findings are not used for the diagnosis of compartment syndrome[11]; however, certain laboratory findings are associated with muscle damage that may occur with compartment syndrome. Serum creatine kinase and myoglobin may be elevated[7,11] and myoglobinuria may also be present.[7] The presence of these laboratory findings indicates the possibility of rhabdomyolysis, a possible complication of the muscle damage from compartment syndrome. Prompt identification and treatment of rhabdomyolysis is necessary. Acute renal failure, acidosis, and fluid and electrolyte imbalances may occur with rhabdomyolysis.[13]

TREATMENT OF ACUTE COMPARTMENT SYNDROME

Prompt surgical fasciotomy is the definitive treatment for acute compartment syndrome. Fasciotomy allows the compartment tissues room to expand without resulting pressure increase.[7] Nursing management of the patient while awaiting surgical treatment should include removal of all restrictive coverings, such as splints or dressings, providing supplementary oxygen, administration of analgesic pain medication, and correction of hypotension.[11] In addition, the affected limb should be kept level with the heart, not elevated or dependent.[11] Postoperatively, the patient will likely require delayed wound closure, and skin grafts may be necessary.[7] Nursing interventions will include maintaining the limb at the level of the heart, strict asepsis during dressing changes, monitoring kidney function, and administration of intravenous (IV) antibiotics.[13]

COMPARTMENT SYNDROME CASE REPORT

BW is a healthy, athletic 20-year-old male admitted following a pedestrian versus motor vehicle collision. He sustained a comminuted fracture of the right tibia and fibula. He was taken from the ED to surgery for an open reduction and external fixation of his injury. On arrival to the orthopedic unit, he is drowsy from sedation, but responds to voice. His vital signs are the following: temperature 96.7°F, pulse 74, respirations 12, and blood pressure 90/62. When transferring BW from the stretcher to the bed, he grimaces and yells out as if in pain; however, he quickly returns to sleep. When awakened, he denies complaint of pain. The nurse completes her initial assessment without waking BW and notices strong posterior tibial and dorsalis pedis pulses bilaterally. Capillary refill is less than 2 seconds and both feet are pink and warm. BW grimaces with pulse assessment on the right, but does not waken.

One hour later, BW awakens with complaint of severe pain to his right lower leg. He rates his pain a 10 on a 1 to 10 scale. The nurse administers 2 mg of morphine IV and reassesses BW's foot. She finds his pulses strong and intact, capillary refill remains less than 2 seconds, and the skin is warm and pink bilaterally. Twenty minutes later, BW's pain is unrelieved by the morphine and he is tearfully rating his pain a 10/10. After administering a second 2-mg dose of morphine without results, the nurse requests additional assessment from the rapid response team (RRT). On arrival, the RRT critical care nurse discovers that BW reports feeling "pins and needles" on the dorsal surface of the right foot. Despite continuing normal vascular assessment, the orthopedic surgeon is notified.

Compartment pressure measurement by the physician revealed elevated compartment pressure and low delta pressure to the anterior compartment of the right lower leg. BW is taken back to the operating room (OR) for an emergency fasciotomy to relieve the compartment pressure. He responds well to the procedure and is discharged home 3 days later with full return of motor and sensory function anticipated.

BW had several risk factors that predisposed him to compartment syndrome. His area of injury is responsible for approximately 40% of compartment syndrome cases.[3] In addition, his age, gender, and activity level are consistent with increased muscle mass, allowing less room for edema within the compartment. BW's low diastolic blood pressure placed him at increased risk of compartment syndrome, because of the role of the arteriovenous gradient in perfusion. Sedation from surgery may have masked his early symptoms of pain, although he did feel increased pain with movement of his extremity. The "Ps" of pallor, pulselessness, paralysis, and poikilothermia are often late findings in compartment syndrome and are associated with significant neurovascular compromise and tissue damage. Pain and paresthesia were important early findings for BW, although these may be difficult to assess in a critically ill or nonverbal patient. Serial assessments and a high index of suspicion in patients at risk are important factors in recognition of acute compartment syndrome.

PATHOPHYSIOLOGY OF FES

FES was first described in 1873[6]; however, the precise cause of the condition is still unclear. Fat emboli are a common occurrence in long-bone and pelvic fractures.[6] It is estimated that 50% to 90% of patients with fracture develop fat in their serum.[6,15] Most of these patients, however, never exhibit signs of FES.[6,15] A small number of cases, however, do go on to develop respiratory, cutaneous, and neurologic symptoms indicative of FES.[6,15] There are 2 theories that address the pathophysiology of FES, the mechanical and biochemical theories:

- Mechanical: Fat globules are released from the site of injury and enter vessels damaged by trauma. They travel through the venous system and enter the arterial system through either a patent foramen ovale or directly from the lungs because of their small size. They cause direct damage when they block vessels in the pulmonary, neurologic, or cutaneous systems.[6,15,16]
- Biochemical: The biochemical theory may be considered on its own, or as an additive process to the mechanical theory.[6] The fat embolized by the injury or fat mobilized by hormonal mediators degrades into free fatty acids and C-reactive protein. This results in capillary leakage, lipid and platelet agglutination, and clot formation.[6,15,16]

FES symptoms typically begin 24 to 72 hours after injury or surgery, giving strength to premise of the biochemical theory that degradation of fat is an important component of this syndrome. In addition, the biochemical theory offers a more reasonable explanation for sources of FES other than trauma, such as pancreatitis, liver disease, and panniculitis.[6]

CLINICAL FINDINGS OF FES

FES typically results in a triad of pulmonary, neurologic, and cutaneous symptoms, as outlined in **Table 2**.

With a history of risk for FES, the characteristic petechiae are considered to be diagnostic for the syndrome.[6,17] However, because rash is not present in all cases and may be the last manifestation to develop, other factors must be considered. Two classification systems to assist in the diagnosis of FES exist and consist of the following criteria:

- Classification of FES, according to Schonfeld and colleagues as cited in DeFeiter et al,[15] consists of weighted scores for the clinical findings of petechiae, diffuse alveolar infiltrates on chest x-ray, hypoxemia, fever, tachycardia, tachypnea, and confusion.
- Classification of FES according to Gurd as cited in DeFeiter et al[15] includes the presence of major and minor criteria. The major criteria include petechiae, respiratory symptoms with bilateral abnormalities on x-ray, and neurologic symptoms

Table 2
Clinical findings of FES

System	Manifestations	Incidence	Onset
Pulmonary	Dyspnea, tachypnea, hypoxemia	75%; 10%–50% progress to respiratory failure	First to develop
Neurologic	Headache, lethargy, agitation, confusion, decreased level of consciousness, seizures, vision changes	80%	After pulmonary symptoms
Cutaneous	Nonpalpable, red-brown, petechiae to the anterior thorax, axilla, and neck	20%–60%	Last to develop

without head trauma. The minor criteria include tachycardia, fever, retinal changes, urinary changes (decreased urine output or lipiduria), thrombocytopenia or anemia, elevated erythrocyte sedimentation rate, and fat in the sputum.

Although both of these classification systems are helpful in identifying findings related to FES, it should be noted that they were developed decades ago, and do not include some of the more sensitive diagnostic testing, such as magnetic resonance imaging (MRI) and computed tomography (CT), that may provide additional support for a diagnosis of FES.[15] The findings for MRI, CT, and other diagnostic testing are described in the next section.

LABORATORY AND DIAGNOSTIC TESTING FOR FES

FES is a diagnosis of exclusion.[18] The clinical findings may mimic those of sepsis, Systemic Inflammatory Response Syndrome (SIRS), pulmonary embolism, or head trauma. Laboratory and diagnostic testing may include the following:

- Arterial blood gas: a Pao_2 of less than 60 mm Hg without evidence of other lung dysfunction and with a history of orthopedic risk factors may indicate FES.[18]
- Serum: blood may be tested for the presence of fat; however, the results do not necessarily indicate FES. Studies have shown that almost all patients with orthopedic injuries consistent with FES risk will be positive for fat in the serum; however, not all of these patients go on to develop FES.[18] Thrombocytopenia, anemia, and an increased erythrocyte sedimentation rate may also be found in some patients with FES.[15]
- Urine: lipiduria may be present,[19] but as with serum lipids, it is not diagnostic for FES. Oliguria or anuria may be present if emboli affect renal function or if cardiac output is affected.[15]
- Sputum: bronchoscopy with lavage may be used to stain macrophages for fat[18,19]; however, this result is also nonspecific, as this is a frequent finding for trauma patients.[18]
- Radiography: chest x-ray may show bilateral infiltrates (resembling acute respiratory distress syndrome), but is normal in many cases.[6,18]
- CT: chest CT often shows a characteristic patchy distribution of "ground glass" opacities and interlobar septal thickening.[6,15] CT of the brain typically does not reveal changes in cases of FES, but may be useful to rule out other causes of central nervous system (CNS) symptoms.[15]
- MRI: MRI of the brain often shows a characteristic "starfield pattern" of multiple, nonconfluent, high-intensity T2 signals. MRI is highly correlated with the degree of clinical neurologic symptoms.[15,18]

TREATMENT OF FES

Prevention of FES is the best option; however, the circumstances that predispose a patient to FES are still not completely understood. It is clear that minimizing disruption to the fracture site, by early splinting for example, will decrease the patient's risk by limiting the fat embolized. A related concept in prevention involves early surgical reduction and fixation of fractures; however, it is unclear if early surgical intervention increases or decreases a patient's risk for FES.[6,18] It is possible that manipulation of the bone during fixation may increase the embolization of fat.[18] It does appear that, if surgical correction is performed, minimizing interosseous pressure during surgery with the use of venting holes decreases the risk of FES.[6,18] The use of prophylactic corticosteroids in patients at risk for FES may also be beneficial; however, studies do not clearly indicate the dosage, timing, or length of steroid therapy that best prevents FES.[6] Standard nursing interventions, such as encouraging coughing and deep breathing and the use of incentive spirometry, may also be helpful in preventing pulmonary complications.[16]

If FES develops, supportive care is the only treatment option available. Although studies have shown some decrease in development of FES with the use of corticosteroids, they are not recommended in the treatment of patients with clinically evident FES. Supportive care includes correction of hypoxia, which often involves mechanical ventilation.[18] Correction of hypovolemia is necessary to prevent shock and worsening CNS ischemia.[15,18] Inotropic medications and pulmonary vasodilators are frequently used.[18] If anemia or thrombocytopenia are present, transfusion with platelets or packed red blood cells may be required.[18] The CNS symptoms involved with FES are typically completely reversible with supportive care.[15]

Although embolization of fat is an almost universal occurrence in a patient with long-bone fracture, the development of FES is a less common complication.[6,15] Most patients who develop FES recover with supportive care. Although mortality rates for FES range from 5% to 15%,[6,15] it should be noted that many of these patients have multiple, traumatic injuries or comorbidities that contribute to the course of their illness.[18]

FES CASE REPORT

JB is a 52-year-old male admitted to the critical care unit following a fall from a ladder while cleaning the gutters at his home. He lives in a remote, rural area and his wife and sons transported him to the local ED in the family vehicle, rather than waiting for an ambulance to arrive. On arrival, he was found to have a right, transverse, midshaft femoral fracture, as well as a fractured clavicle and 2 fractured ribs. He was alert and oriented, and his vital signs were stable. He was taken to the OR for intramedullary nailing of the femur. He arrives to the unit in stable condition, and is anticipated to be transferred to the orthopedic floor the following day.

During the morning, it is noted that JB's respiratory rate has increased from 14 to 20. His SpO$_2$ has decreased from 100% on room air to 94% on room air and he is placed on 2 LPM oxygen by nasal cannula, with a corresponding increase in SpO$_2$ to 96%. He is encouraged to cough and deep breath and shown how to splint his chest to minimize discomfort. JB's wife arrives and, after visiting with him for a few moments, comes to the nurses' station to ask why her husband is "not making sense." On reassessment, the nurse notes that JB's Glasgow Coma Scale score has decreased from 15 to 13. JB is drowsy and confused, and his SpO$_2$ has decreased to 90% on oxygen at 2 LPM. His respiratory rate has increased to 22 and his heart rate is 105 and blood pressure is 126/72. His lung sounds are clear bilaterally. The physician is notified and the respiratory therapist is consulted. JB's hypoxia and tachypnea worsen, and he is placed on a 100% non-rebreather and a stat chest x-ray and arterial blood gas (ABG) are ordered. JB's chest x-ray is unchanged from his baseline, and his ABG is pH 7.38, Pco$_2$ 35 mm Hg, and Pao$_2$ 72 mm Hg. Petechiae are noted on JB's chest and axilla.

A decision is made to intubate and mechanically ventilate JB to support his respiratory function and maintain adequate oxygenation. An arterial line is placed to evaluate ABGs and hemodynamic status. Supportive care is provided for JB and he is extubated 3 days later. His neurologic status returns to baseline within 5 days and he is discharged to a rehabilitation facility 1 week after admission. JB's long-bone fracture, the lack of stabilization at the time of injury, and the surgical procedure to repair his injury all predisposed him to fat emboli. The presence of fat in the circulatory system is common in this type of injury, but does not always result in the respiratory, neurologic, and cutaneous symptoms associated with FES. In the case of JB, his tachypnea and increasing hypoxia were early signs of FES. The neurologic symptoms he experienced are common findings in FES that typically resolve completely. MRI and CT would have been helpful to confirm the diagnosis of FES and rule out other sources of respiratory and neurologic symptoms; however, these were not available. The petechial rash JB developed is characteristic of FES, but not present in all cases. Prompt recognition of FES and early supportive care will assist the patient to a full recovery.

SUMMARY

This article highlights 2 important complications of fracture: acute compartment syndrome and FES. FES is most commonly associated with long-bone and pelvic fracture, whereas acute compartment syndrome is often associated with tibia or forearm fracture. The onset of both of these complications may be difficult to assess in the nonverbal patient or the patient with multiple trauma. Careful, serial assessment of the patient with fracture is necessary to recognize and treat these complications promptly. Early treatment and supportive care are crucial to positive outcomes for patients with complications of fracture.

REFERENCES

1. Hoyert DL, Xu J. Deaths: preliminary data for 2011. National Vital Statistics Report; 61. Available at: www.cdc.gov. Accessed October 15, 2012.
2. Centers for Disease Control and Prevention. Sports, recreation, and exercise. Available at: www.cdc.gov/injury. Accessed October 15, 2012.
3. Menkes JS. Initial evaluation and management of orthopedic injuries. In: Tintinalli JE, Stapczynski JS, Ma OJ, et al, editors. Tintinalli's emergency medicine: a comprehensive study guide. 7th edition. New York: McGraw Hill; 2011. p. 1783–96.
4. Buetler A, Stephens MB. General principles of fracture management: bone healing and fracture description. Available at: http://www.uptodate.com. Accessed September 10, 2012.
5. Morin RJ, Swan KG, Tan V. Acute forearm compartment syndrome secondary to local arterial injury after penetrating trauma. J Trauma 2009;66(4):989–93.
6. Weinhouse GL. Fat embolism syndrome. Available at: http://www.uptodate.com. Accessed October 15, 2012.
7. Haller PR. Compartment syndrome. In: Tintinalli JE, Stapczynski JS, Ma OJ, et al, editors. Tintinalli's emergency medicine: a comprehensive study guide. 7th edition. New York: McGraw Hill; 2011. p. 1880–4.
8. Morton PG, Fontaine DK. Trauma. In: Morton, Fontaine, editors. Essentials of critical care nursing. Philadelphia: Lippincott Williams & Wilkins; 2013. p. 470–86.
9. Kosir R, Moore FA, Selby JH, et al. Acute lower extremity compartment syndrome (ALECS) screening protocol in critically ill trauma patients. J Trauma 2007;63(2):268–75.
10. Wright E. Neurovascular impairment and compartment syndrome. Paediatr Nurs 2009;21(3):26–9.
11. Stracciolini A, Hammerberg EM. Acute compartment syndrome of the extremities. Available at: http://www.uptodate.com. Accessed October 15, 2012.
12. Johnson-Walker E, Hardcastle J. Neurovascular assessment in the critically ill patient. Nurs Crit Care 2011;16(4):170–7.

13. Bongiovanni MS, Bradley SL, Kelley DM. Orthopedic trauma: critical care nursing issues. Crit Care Nurs Q 2005;28(1):60–71.

14. Tousignant-Laflamme Y, Bourgault P, Gelinas C, et al. Assessing pain behaviors in healthy subjects using the critical-care pain observation tool (CPOT): a pilot study. J Pain 2010;11(10):983–7.

15. De Feiter PW, Van Hooft MA, Beets-Tan RG, et al. Fat embolism syndrome: yes or no? J Trauma 2007;63(2):429–31.

16. Gore T, Lacey S. Bone up on fat embolism syndrome. Nursing 2005;35:32hn1–4.

17. Powers KA, Talbot LA. Fat embolism syndrome after femur fracture with intramedullary nailing: case report. Am J Crit Care 2011;20:264–7.

18. Galaway U, Tetzlaff JE, Helfand R. Acute fatal fat embolism syndrome in bilateral total knee arthroplasty: a review of the fat embolism syndrome. Internet J Anesthesiol 2009;19(2):1–14.

19. Cothren CC, Moore EE, Vanderheiden T, et al. Occam's razor is a double-edged sword: concomitant pulmonary embolism and fat embolism syndrome. J Trauma 2008;65(6):1558–60.

Travel-Related Illness

Carol C. Ziegler, DNP, FNP, RN

KEYWORDS

- Global health • Travel health • Travel illness • Travel guidelines • Global diseases
- Disease prevention • PTHA • Destination-based risk assessment

KEY POINTS

- The key to managing travel-related illness is prevention.
- Pretravel health assessment is vital in assuring safe travel for all persons, especially those with chronic conditions.
- Using the destination-based risk assessment, the nurse can help patients make contingency plans for the treatment of illnesses and diseases while abroad.
- Travel-related infections are typically transmitted via blood, soil, insects, or other vectors, such as livestock, sexual contact, air, or water.
- Traveling while pregnant presents a unique list of considerations.
- There are multiple diseases that are more prevalent in countries other than the United States that warrant special consideration for American and Canadian travelers.

Worldwide, the number of people traveling internationally has ballooned to 935 million in 2010 alone.[1,2] Research in travel medicine has grown tremendously in the past 10 years, and the prevalence of specialized travel clinics is increasing. As international travel becomes more common and more affordable, nurses increasingly provide care for persons embarking on or returning from travel abroad. Many patients seek care just before departure rather than visiting a specialty travel clinic. With global travel, nurses should be aware of the potential travel-related illnesses with which their patients might present on return from foreign travel. Additionally, for patients with chronic diseases, it is imperative that nurses have resources for accessing destination-specific information for patients before their departure to help prevent their patients from contracting diseases that might make their underlying conditions worse.

In addition to providing care to traveling patients, nurses themselves are increasingly involved in health service projects abroad. Providing health care in the global arena presents a unique set of health risks and destination-based exposures. Having knowledge and a clear understanding of the basic elements of caring for the international traveler, including the pretravel health assessment (PTHA), the destination-based risk assessment (DBRA), and the prevention of common travel-related

Vanderbilt University School of Nursing, 345 Frist Hall, 461 21st Avenue South, Nashville, TN 37240, USA
E-mail address: carol.c.ziegler@vanderbilt.edu

Crit Care Nurs Clin N Am 25 (2013) 333–340
http://dx.doi.org/10.1016/j.ccell.2013.02.015
0899-5885/13/$ – see front matter © 2013 Elsevier Inc. All rights reserved.

illnesses, is essential. Practice guidelines are constantly being revised and updated, and it is important to keep current in today's global health care milieu.

BEFORE THE TRIP: ANTICIPATORY GUIDANCE

The growing burden of global infectious disease leads the prudent nurse to recognize anticipatory guidance as a critical first step in mitigating health risks associated with international travel. Because of the evidence that few patients seek care before travelling abroad, it is prudent for nurses to inform patients at routine visits, before initiating travel plans, that they should seek pretravel care at least a month in advance, if possible, or as soon as possible if they intend to travel abroad in the future. This anticipatory guidance is the first step in mitigating risk for patients and local communities. Recent outbreaks of measles and dengue fever in the United States could have been prevented had persons traveling abroad taken precautions before traveling and returning.[3,4] Anticipatory guidance is important for all travelers, especially those with chronic diseases and conditions.

THE PTHA

Although anticipatory guidance makes patients aware of the need to seek health care before travel, the PTHA is often the first step beyond routine primary care in providing care to the international traveler. The PTHA is a patient-specific review of travel-related risks; purpose of travel and basic itinerary; current immunization status; current health status, including medications, chronic conditions, and completion of regular health maintenance; and assessment of any concerns patients may have about their health or travel plans.

Overview of General Travel-Related Risks

International travel poses general health risks for all individuals that should be discussed with patients. Patients who succumb to these risks are often hospitalized. Air travel has been linked to deep vein thromboses (DVT) and airborne infections. Bodily injury caused by crime, civil unrest, and even road accidents in host countries are all potential risks that international travelers may experience. Differences in access to medical care abroad should be assessed and discussed with patients based on the risks associated with their destination. Personal behavioral choices, such as alcohol and drug use and sexual behavior, and the risk of contracting and spreading sexually transmitted infections should be discussed. Self-care and management of any chronic conditions, such as diabetes, hypertension, or mental illness, should be assessed and discussed with travelers at the pretravel visit. Increasing awareness of potential health consequences rather than alarming patients should be the clear motive in these discussions.

Purpose of Travel

The purpose of travel, whether leisure, business, or health service work, provides insight into the potential risks to be encountered by patients. Patients traveling for business purposes may plan a longer duration of stay, and the length of travel is strongly associated with the overall health risk and risk for contracting infectious diseases.[5] Persons traveling for service work are at increased risk of exposure to local infectious diseases while providing care in areas that may not have barrier methods available for preventing blood-borne infections. Persons traveling for leisure to visit family may have lowered vigilance of malaria prophylaxis or food- and water-borne illness prevention strategies, believing incorrectly that they have continuous immunity from childhood exposures.

Current Immunization Status

It is critical to get an accurate assessment of the current immunization status at the PTHA, an opportune time to ensure that patients are up to date on routine vaccinations. For optimal efficiency, patients should be informed of the need to bring all vaccination records to the visit at the time they schedule the appointment. If patients present for the visit with inadequate lead time to obtain immunoglobulin titer results for immunity, it is prudent to go ahead and administer needed vaccines in the absence of accurate health records. Routine vaccines include hepatitis A and B, tetanus/diphtheria/pertussis, human papillomavirus, measles/mumps/rubella, varicella, pneumococcal, meningococcal, zoster, and flu and should be updated before travel according to current guidelines. Annually updated immunization schedules for children and adults may be found at the Centers for Disease Control and Prevention (CDC) Web site (www.cdc.gov/vaccines/schedules/index.html). The need for further destination-specific vaccines is discussed in the DBRA portion of this article.

Current Health Status

Pretravel health status is thoroughly assessed at the PTHA. This assessment provides the clinician with baseline information if patients return with an illness and alerts the provider to additional risk that patients may be exposed to beyond those normally associated with international travel. Past medical history should be reviewed and updated, including any risk factors for chronic disease. Control of any preexisting conditions, such as allergies, psychological illnesses, cardiovascular disease, diabetes, immune-mediated illnesses, and intestinal illnesses, should be assessed with a thorough history and physical examination, augmented with any necessary laboratory tests. All current medications, doses, and schedules should be reviewed and updated, and patients should be provided with an adequate supply of needed medications for the duration of their travel.

Nurses should discuss strategies to optimize the management of any chronic conditions while abroad, from ensuring adequate supply of medications to managing time zone changes and food/water considerations while traveling. The need for medical documentation of any medical devices or medications should be assessed and provided to patients for air travel or navigating local customs authorities. Patients with chronic conditions are well advised to carry a summarized copy of their medical record while traveling abroad in case of an emergency.

DBRA

Once the current health of patients has been assessed, the clinician should conduct a DBRA to determine what specific health risks patients may face according to their specific destination. Nurses should review the CDC travel Web site for each destination at the time of the visit because information changes frequently. Resources for providers are discussed in detail in a later section. The provider should assess the time until departure, method of travel, presence or absence of travel companions, purpose of travel and length of stay, accommodations, need for additional vaccinations, and major health risks associated with the destination. Increased risk for travel-related illness may be affected by destination, length of stay, itinerary, purpose of travel, preexisting medical conditions, and personal behavior.[6]

Travel-related infections are typically transmitted via blood, soil, insects, or other vectors, such as livestock, sexual contact, air, or water. An exhaustive list of destination-specific travel-related infections may be found at the CDC travel Web site (http://wwwnc.cdc.gov/travel/destinations/list) and additional destination-specific resources are provided at the end of the article in tabular format. On review of the infections associated with international travel, an incomplete but comprehensive list includes anthrax, brucellosis, cholera, dengue fever, typhoid, *Giardia*, flu, meningitis, hemorrhagic fevers, Hantavirus, viral hepatitis (A, B, C, and E), plague, tuberculosis, malaria, traveler's diarrhea, and sexually transmitted infections. The most common infection associated with travel is traveler's diarrhea, affecting 30% to 70% of all international travelers.[7]

Mitigating Travel-Related Health Risks

Once the PTHA and DBRA have been completed and risks and requirements have been clearly identified, the clinician creates the pretravel health plan to mitigate destination-specific travel-related health risks. This plan typically includes instructions and preparation strategies for the management of any chronic diseases; administration of any required and/or suggested vaccinations; counseling on strategies to avoid contracting illness; and provision of prophylactic therapy for any likely infections, such as traveler's diarrhea and malaria.

Patients should be educated about avoiding general risks, such as practicing safer sex and avoiding alcohol or drug intoxication. Strategies for additional risk avoidance, such as risk for road accidents or crime, would include advice such as minimizing nighttime travel, traveling in groups, and maintaining awareness of surroundings. Keeping identification and travel documents on your person at all times and separated from cash is wise in the event of theft.

Vaccines

In addition to the routine vaccines described previously, commonly required pretravel vaccines may include those against typhoid, yellow fever, rabies, cholera, and Japanese encephalitis. A recent study revealed that a retrospective analysis of patients seen at travel clinics most commonly received hepatitis A and typhoid vaccines.[6] Yellow fever vaccine is required for entry into many countries and is only available to be administered by certified providers. Therefore, if you are not a certified yellow fever vaccine provider, it is critical to advise patients of the need for this vaccine and provide information for where to obtain it in your local community.

Blood-borne illnesses and sexually transmitted infections

Discuss safer sex practices with all patients, and advise consistent condom use if they are sexually active. A general discussion of avoidance of common sexually transmitted infections, such as human immunodeficiency virus (HIV), hepatitis B, syphilis, gonorrhea, and *Chlamydia*, should be discussed with patients. Patients should avoid contact with blood and should be educated about universal precautions.

Soil, food, and waterborne sources

Educate the traveler on general strategies to avoid common infections like hepatitis A, typhoid fever, and cholera, such as avoiding contact with contaminated water by only drinking boiled or bottled water, avoid ingesting peelings of fruits and vegetables, and avoid food sold by street vendors. Travelers should be aware that even eating food off of plates washed in contaminated water might make them ill. The advice *boil it, peel it, or forget it* is prudent; but patients may follow these tenets and still contract illness from locally prepared foods. Eating only hot foods may mitigate some risk of food-borne illness. Swimming in contaminated water should be avoided.

Animal sources

Exposure to pathogens from animals from bites, direct contact, or ingesting meat or milk can be avoided by avoiding contact with domestic and wild animals. Unpasteurized milk and dairy products and undercooked meat should be avoided. Careful hand washing after any contact with animals and making sure to wear hard-soled shoes may also protect the traveler from zoonoses. Rabies is discussed in the following section.

Airborne infections

Hand washing, good respiratory hygiene, and avoiding contact with infected persons should be discussed with patients. Patients traveling to areas endemic for tuberculosis should be advised to be tested at some point soon after their return. Vaccinating patients against influenza before their departure may prevent influenza infection.

Vector-borne infections

Vectors, such as mosquitoes, flies, and ticks, are common sources of travel-related illness. Travelers should be counseled on strategies to avoid bites. Chemoprophylaxis against malaria, vaccination against yellow fever, and consistent use of insecticide-treated bed nets, specifically N,N-diethyl-3-methylbenzamine (DEET), help to minimize risk. During the day, travelers should be advised to minimize exposed skin to avoid bites and complete daily self-checks for ticks as needed.

Recent Updates and New Evidence

In the past 2 years, new recommendations have been created relating to several vaccine-preventable diseases, yellow fever, rabies postexposure prophylaxis (PEP), malaria, and new strains of antibiotic-resistant bacteria. These new guidelines are discussed later.

Yellow fever

Many countries are tightening enforcement of yellow fever vaccination requirements, and patients traveling to these countries should be advised to ensure that they have the yellow fever vaccination certificate with them while traveling. Patients should be aware that even when traveling through these municipalities to get to a final destination, proof of yellow fever vaccination status might be required to move through customs enforcement and security. The World Health Organization (WHO) and the CDC released new country-specific yellow fever vaccine recommendations in 2011 and 2012.[7,8] Providers should review this information frequently and advise patients based on destination exposure risk, country entry requirements, and individual risk factors for contracting yellow fever or reacting to the vaccine.[9]

Rabies

Rabies exposure in travelers is more common than you may think, and published case reports of travelers exposed to rabies while visiting Indonesia and Austria were found in the literature.[10,11] Travelers from countries requiring immunization of household pets often assume incorrectly that dogs or other animals they may encounter abroad are also vaccinated. Remind patients that many countries do not require rabies vaccination of common household pets, so approaching any animal may be dangerous. In 2010, the Advisory Committee on Immunization Practices released new guidelines for PEP regimens against rabies, which recommends 4 doses of rabies vaccine for PEP.[12] However, access to this vaccine may be limited in many countries abroad, and travelers should be advised to avoid contact with animals.

Malaria

One of the greatest risks to international travelers is malaria, and malaria prophylaxis is often the sole factor prompting patients to seek pretravel care. All patients traveling to malaria-endemic areas should receive malaria prophylaxis. Many providers prescribe doxycycline for malaria prophylaxis incorrectly because resistance to doxycycline is increasing in many endemic regions. An up-to-date list of malaria-endemic destinations as well as the presence or absence of resistant malaria strains and recommended medications for chemoprophylaxis from the CDC may be found at http://www.cdc.gov/malaria/.[7] This information should be checked frequently for updates.

Antibiotic resistance

Antibiotic resistance is a growing global threat. Failure to adhere to evidence-based prescribing practices is root of this problem. A literature search for travel-related antibiotic resistance patterns reveals that traveler's diarrhea is most often linked to antibiotic resistance. Specifically with regard to traveler's diarrhea, the most common travel-related illness, resistance to the most commonly prescribed medications, fluoroquinolones and azithromycin, is increasingly reported.[13] However, at present, the CDC still recommends advising patients to self-treat with a fluoroquinolone (http://wwwnc.cdc.gov/travel/yellowbook/2012/chapter-16-the-pre-travel-consultation/travelers-diarrhea.htm).

The Pregnant Traveler

Traveling internationally while pregnant presents a unique set of risks, and all pregnant persons seeking pretravel care should discuss their travel plans and risks with their nurse midwife or obstetrician before departure. In addition to consultation with her midwife or obstetric provider, the PTHA of pregnant patients should involve a thorough discussion of recommended vaccinations and their safety, avoidance of food, air, soil, water, and vector-borne illnesses specific to the destination, and malaria prophylaxis if indicated. Keep in mind that malaria, yellow fever, tuberculosis, rubella, typhoid, dengue fever, HIV, and hepatitis infections can occur in utero.[14] The CDC's recommendations for vaccinating pregnant travelers can be found at http://wwwnc.cdc.gov/travel/yellowbook/2012/chapter-6-advising-travelers-with-specific-needs/pregnant-travelers.htm. Patients must be counseled that the safety profiles of some commonly recommended vaccinations, such as yellow fever and typhoid fever, are unknown in pregnancy and that live, attenuated vaccines are contraindicated in pregnancy.

Air travel

According to the American College of Obstetricians and Gynecologists, healthy pregnant women may travel safely up to 36 weeks' gestation. However, patients are well advised to check with specific airlines regarding requirements and limitations for travel in pregnancy. Air travel has not been proven to be a risk factor for pregnant women, but the risk for DVT is increased in pregnancy because of hypercoagulability.[15] Mitigating risks for pregnant women who must travel internationally should include counseling regarding exercise during air travel, especially on flights of 8 hours or more. To minimize the risk of DVT, maintaining hydration, despite increased urination, and walking every 2 hours are recommended strategies.

Malaria

All pregnant women traveling to malaria-endemic areas are at an increased risk of contracting malaria, but this risk is increased slightly if they are primigravida. They should be informed that gestational malaria increases the risk for preterm birth and low birthweight as well as spontaneous abortion and stillbirths.[14] The best prevention strategies include minimizing the number of mosquito bites with consistent use of DEET-treated bed nets and oral chemoprophylaxis with mefloquine or chloroquine (thought to be safe in the second and third trimesters). Women should be counseled that although safety of these medications is unknown in the first trimester, it is generally accepted practice that the risk of harm from mefloquine to the first-trimester fetus is lower than the risk of harm from malaria[14]; the CDC recently released guidelines recommending that mefloquine be used as a prophylaxis for and treatment of malaria in all trimesters (http://www.cdc.gov/malaria/new_info/2011/mefloquine_pregnancy.html).

Travel Warnings and Conflict Areas

Mitigating the risks of travel in conflict zones is outside of the scope of this article. However, advise all patients traveling abroad to check with the US State Department regarding any recent travel warnings related to their destination (http://travel.state.gov/travel/cis_pa_tw/cis_pa_tw_1168.html). Advise travelers to register with the US State Department before departure if they are traveling to an area with warnings in place and to maintain copies of all travel and identification documents, passports, and health records with contacts in the United States.

Resources for Providers

As travel medicine grows, more information on evidence-based care becomes available. New knowledge is accompanied by rapid changes in the global environment related to travel patterns, exposure risks, and emerging and reemerging infectious diseases and antibiotic resistance patterns. Change is so rapid that by the time of printing, this article will be partially out of date. Providers caring for international travelers must rapidly incorporate emerging evidence into their clinical tool kit. A list of reliable and regularly updated resources available for both providers and patients is outlined in **Table 1**.

The CDC, the WHO, and the US State Department have up-to-date information on travel warnings, recommendations, and requirements. Also, the Infectious Disease Society of America (IDSA) and the International Society of Travel Medicine (ISTM)

Table 1
Resources for health information on international travel

Organization	Source	Information
CDC	*The Yellow Book* http://wwwnc.cdc.gov/travel	Health information for international travel
WHO	*The Green Book* http://www.who.int/ith/en/	International health regulation guidelines for travel
US State Department	www.state.gov/travel	Travel warnings, country-specific entry requirements, required immunizations
IDSA	http://www.idsociety.org/IDSA_Practice_Guidelines	Practice guidelines for international travelers
ISID	www.promedmail.org	Reports outbreaks and emerging diseases
ISTM	http://www.istm.org	Updates on emerging travel-related illnesses
US OTTI	http://tinet.ita.doc.gov	Current travel patterns into and from the United States
Health map	http://www.healthmap.org/en/	Maps global infectious diseases

have up-to-date guidelines and advice for practitioners caring for this unique population. The International Society for Infectious Diseases (ISID) has a Web site (www. promedmail.org) that details the latest disease outbreaks and alerts worldwide. For data on international travel to and from the United States, the Office of Travel and Tourism Industries (OTTI) in the Department of Commerce is the best source of information. As global travel becomes more accessible to more individuals, well-informed nurses using evidence-based practice will be critical players in protecting communities from emerging infectious diseases.

REFERENCES

1. World Health Organization. International travel and health. Available at: http:// www.who.int/ith. Accessed September 14, 2012.
2. World Tourism Organization. Facts and figures. Available at: http://www.unwto. org/facts/menu. Accessed October 2, 2012.
3. Centers for Disease Control and Prevention. Locally acquired dengue-Key West, Florida, 2009-2010. MMWR Morb Mortal Wkly Rep 2010;59:577–81.
4. Centers for Disease Control and Prevention. Measles: Untied States, January-may 20, 2011. MMWR Morb Mortal Wkly Rep 2011;60:666–8.
5. Chen L, Wilson M, Davis X, et al. Illness in long-term travelers visiting geo-sentinel clinics. Emerg Infect Dis 2009;15(11):1773–82.
6. LaRocque R, Sowmya R, Lee J, et al. Global TravEpiNet: a national consortium of clinics providing care to international travelers – analysis of demographic characteristics, travel destinations and pretravel healthcare of high-risk US international travelers, 2009-2011. Clin Infect Dis 2012;54(4):455–62.
7. Centers for Disease Control. 2012. Available at: http://wwwnc.cdc.gov/travel/ yellowbook/2012/chapter-2-the-pre-travel-consultation/travelers-diarrhea.htm. Accessed September 9, 2012.
8. WHO. 2011.
9. LaRocque. 2011.
10. Gautret P, Lim P, Shaw M, et al. Rabies postexposure prophylaxis in travelers returning from Bali, Indonesia, November 2008 to March 2010. Clin Microbiol Infect 2011;17:445–7.
11. Strauss R, Granz A, Wasserman M, et al. A human case of travel-related rabies in Austria, September, 2004. Euro Surveill 2005;10:225–6.
12. Rupprecht C, Briggs D, Brown C, et al. Use of a reduced (4-dose) vaccine schedule for postexposure prophylaxis to prevent human rabies: recommendations of the Advisory Committee on Immunization Practices. MMWR Recomm Rep 2010;59:1–9.
13. Ouyang-Latimer L, Jafri S, VanTassel L, et al. In vitro antimicrobial susceptibility of bacterial enteropathogens isolated from international travelers to Mexico, Guatemala and India from 2006 to 2008. Antimicrob Agents Chemother 2011; 55:874–8.
14. McGovern L, Boyce T, Fischer P. Congenital infections associated with international travel during pregnancy. J Travel Med 2007;14(2):117–28. Accessed September 20, 2012.
15. American College of Obstetricians and Gynecologists (ACOG). Air travel during pregnancy. Obstet Gynecol 2001;98(6):1187–8.

Index

Note: Page numbers of article titles are in **boldface** type.

Crit Care Nurs Clin N Am 25 (2013) 341–350
http://dx.doi.org/10.1016/S0899-5885(13)00038-5
0899-5885/13/$ – see front matter © 2013 Elsevier Inc. All rights reserved.

Moving?

Make sure your subscription moves with you!

To notify us of your new address, find your **Clinics Account Number** (located on your mailing label above your name), and contact customer service at:

Email: journalscustomerservice-usa@elsevier.com

800-654-2452 (subscribers in the U.S. & Canada)
314-447-8871 (subscribers outside of the U.S. & Canada)

Fax number: 314-447-8029

Elsevier Health Sciences Division
Subscription Customer Service
3251 Riverport Lane
Maryland Heights, MO 63043

*To ensure uninterrupted delivery of your subscription, please notify us at least 4 weeks in advance of move.

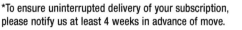

Printed and bound by CPI Group (UK) Ltd, Croydon, CR0 4YY

03/10/2024

01040439-0002